Reviving

An Effective Guide And Cookbook For Stomach Ulcers with over 150 Plant-Base-Belly-Soothing Recipes For Old And Newly Diagnosed

© **Luckas Thomas (BSc, RD.)**

All rights reserved. No parts of this publication may be reproduced, stored in retrieval system, or transmitted in any form or by any means, electronic, mechanical, photocopying, recording, or otherwise, without the prior written permission of the author.

TABLE OF CONTENTS

Introduction 1
   Symptoms Of Stomach Ulcers 3
   NSAID Drugs And Stomach Ulcers 5
   Types of Stomach Of Ulcers 6
   Treatment 8
   Diagnosis 8
   Home Relief For Stomach Ulcers 12
   Risky Factors Of Developing Ulcers 13
   Ways Of Preventing Ulcers 18

Food Preparation And Meal Planning For Stomach Ulcers. (Both For Adults And Children) 18
   How To Feed Especially When You Have Stomach Ulcers 19

MEAL IDEAS FOR STOMACH ULCERS 22
   FODMAP Food 24
   Mealtime Tips 25

PLANT-BASE-BELLY-SOOTHING RECIPES FOR OLD AND NEWLY DIAGNOSED 27
   Breakfasts Recipes 28
   Lunches Recipes 50
   Dinners Recipes 77
   Snacks and Desserts Recipes 129

Introduction

Stomach ulcers, also known as gastric ulcers, are painful sores on the lining of the stomach. Peptic ulcer disease manifests itself as stomach ulcers. Any ulcer that affects both the stomach and the small intestines is referred to as a peptic ulcer. Stomach ulcers develop as the thick layer of mucus that protects the stomach from digestive juices thins. This causes the digestive acids to erode at the stomach tissues, resulting in an ulcer.

The stomach secretes a powerful acid that aids digestion and protects against microbes. It also secretes a thick layer of mucus to shield the body's tissues from this acid. If the mucus layer wears away and stops working properly, the acid can damage stomach tissue, resulting in an ulcer.

One out of every ten people in Western countries will develop a stomach or small intestine ulcer at some stage in their lives.

Stomach ulcers are more common in people over the age of 50. A stomach ulcer can occur at any age, but it is much less common in children. Children are at a higher risk if their parents smoke. While stomach ulcers are easily treated, they can become serious if not treated properly.

Causes of Stomach Ulcers

One of the following usually triggers stomach ulcers:

- Infection with the Helicobacter pylori bacterium (H. pylori)

- Usage of nonsteroidal anti-inflammatory medications (NSAIDs) such as aspirin, ibuprofen, or naproxen for an extended period of time

- A disorder known as Zollinger-Ellison syndrome can cause stomach and intestinal ulcers in rare cases by increasing the body's acid output. This disease is believed to be responsible for less than 1% of all peptic ulcers.

NSAIDs, a type of pain reliever, may increase the risk of stomach ulcers.

The following are some of the less common causes of stomach ulcers:

Excess stomach acidity, also known as hyperacidity, can occur for a variety of reasons, including biology, smoking, stress, and certain foods.

Symptoms Of Stomach Ulcers

Stomach ulcers are associated with a variety of symptoms. The severity of the symptoms is determined by the extent of the ulcer.

A burning feeling or pain in the center of your abdomen between your chest and belly button is the most common symptom. When your stomach is empty, the pain is usually more intense, and it can last anywhere from a few minutes to several hours.

Ulcers can also cause the following signs and symptoms:

- Loss of weight
- Not feeling hungry because of pain
- Vomiting or nausea
- Bloating
- Feeling easily full
- Acid reflux or burping
- Heartburn, which is a burning sensation in the chest)
- Tiredness, shortness of breath, and paler skin are all signs of anemia
- Dark, tarry stools
- Bloody Vomit

If you have the signs of a stomach ulcer, consult your doctor. Even if the pain is minor, ulcers will worsen if not treated. Ulcers that bleed profusely can be fatal.

Eating, drinking, or having antacids may lessen pain.

Some stomach ulcers go undetected because they don't cause indigestion. These ulcers are less common, and they are usually discovered after the ulcer has begun to bleed. A break in the stomach wall may be caused by certain ulcers. This is referred to as perforation, and it is a potentially fatal disease.

Symptoms of a stomach ulcer can change over time and be difficult to detect.

Dietary Changes
Changes in diet can help prevent stomach ulcers from forming.

People who are at risk of stomach ulcers should eat more of the following nutrients:

Fruits and vegetables: A diverse diet rich in fruits and vegetables is important for maintaining a healthy digestive tract lining. These foods are high in antioxidants, inhibit acid secretion, and have anti-inflammatory and cytoprotective effects. According to a 2017 report, these are all crucial factors in preventing and treating ulcers.

Dietary fiber: reduces the risk of stomach ulcers in people who eat a high-fiber diet.

Probiotic: yogurt, for example, contains active bacterial material and may help to minimize Helicobacter pylori (H. pylori) infection. Probiotics have been shown to help with indigestion symptoms as well as antibiotic side effects..

Vitamin C: This effective antioxidant may aid in the eradication of H. pylori, especially when taken in small doses over a long period. Vitamin C is abundant in fruits, legumes, and vegetables such as oranges and tomatoes.

Zinc: This micronutrient is essential for wound healing and maintaining a healthy immune system. Zinc is abundant in oysters, lettuce, and beef.

Selenium: This can lower the risk of infection complications and speed up the healing process. Brazil nuts, yellow fin tuna, and halibut are recommended due to their high selenium content,

Avoiding alcohol and caffeine, which both cause the body to produce more gastric acid, may also help reduce the risk. This can contribute to stomach ulcers.

Instead of focusing solely on food, it is important to use nutritional choices to endorse a treatment plan for the best results.

NSAID Drugs And Stomach Ulcers

The use of NSAIDs, or nonsteroidal anti-inflammatory drugs, increases the risk of stomach ulcers. Aspirin and ibuprofen are the two most well-known NSAIDs.

If the medications are taken in high doses or on a daily basis, the risk of ulcers increases. Stronger NSAIDs, such as those that require a prescription, are more likely to cause stomach ulcers than over-the-counter NSAIDs (OTC).

People should always read labels and consult a pharmacist or a doctor if they have any questions or doubts about painkillers. They may suggest acetaminophen as an alternative.

Types of Stomach Of Ulcers

Peptic ulcers come in many different forms. Stomach ulcers are one of them.

There are two main types: Esophageal and duodenal ulcers. Duodenal ulcers occur in the uppermost region of the small intestine, known as the duodenum, and esophageal ulcers occur within the esophagus.

Ulcers have identical features, but their position in the body distinguishes them.

Finding out where and when the symptoms start is one way to say whether you have a gastric or duodenal ulcer. The time between meals can aggravate an ulcer in some people. Others can experience pain when they eat.

However, the precise location of the pain does not necessarily correspond to the location of the ulcer. Pain can be felt in some cases. This means that a person can experience pain in a location beyond the ulcer itself.

Some signs and symptoms include

- Nausea
- Vomiting
- Bloating

Many ulcer signs, according to digestive specialists, are caused by bleeding. However, almost 75% of people with gastric or duodenal ulcers have no symptoms.

If you have serious symptoms, they may include:

- Blood in your stool, or stool that appears black or tarry
- Breathing difficulties
- Experiencing dizziness or losing consciousness
- Blood in the vomit
- Shortness of breath when doing something active
- Tiredness

If you have abdominal pain and all of the above signs, see a doctor right away.

Treatment

If your doctor suspects you have a stomach ulcer, they may try to treat it by:

Changing the form of painkiller if NSAIDs are suspected as the cause. If H. pylori bacteria is suspected as the cause, try the "test-and-treat" approach..Stomach ulcers can be treated by shielding the ulcer from acid as it heals until the cause has been eliminated. The following are examples of drugs that a doctor might prescribe:

- Proton pump inhibitors (PPI) that block acid-producing cells
- H2-receptor antagonists, which prevent the stomach from producing excess acid
- Drugs that protect the stomach lining, such as Pepto-Bismol.
- Antacids or alginate. These can be purchased over-the-counter or on the internet.

After treatment, symptoms usually go away quickly. However, if the ulcer is caused by an H. pylori infection, the treatment should be continued. During therapy, you should stop consuming alcohol, smoking cigarettes, and eating any trigger foods.

Diagnosis

Your symptoms and the seriousness of your ulcer will determine your diagnosis and treatment options. Your doctor will examine your medical history, symptoms, and any prescription or over-the-counter drugs you're taking to determine whether you have a stomach ulcer.

A blood, stool, or breath test may be ordered to rule out H. pylori infection. A breath test requires you to drink a clear liquid and then breathe into a bag that is then sealed. If H. pylori is present, the carbon dioxide levels in the breath sample will be higher than normal.

Other tests and procedures used to diagnose stomach ulcers include:

- **Barium swallow**: You drink a thick white liquid (barium) that coats your upper gastrointestinal tract and helps your doctor see your stomach and small intestine on X-rays.
- **Endoscopy (EGD):** A thin, lighted tube is inserted through your mouth and into the stomach and the first part of the small intestine. This test is used to look for ulcers, bleeding, and any tissue that looks abnormal.
- **Endoscopic biopsy**: A piece of stomach tissue is removed so it can be analyzed in a lab.

Surgical Procedures

Surgery could be a choice in some cases. If the ulcer returns, does not heal, bleeds, or prevents food from leaving the stomach, for example.

Surgical procedures include:

- Removing the ulcer
- Tying off blood vessels that are bleeding
- Using tissue from a different location to sew onto the ulcer
- Cutting the nerve that influences the development of stomach acid. Stomach ulcer complications such as bleeding or perforation are uncommon. Any of these issues necessitates immediate medical attention.

The type of treatment you receive will be determined by the cause of your ulcer. The majority of ulcers can be treated with a prescription from your doctor, but surgery may be needed in extreme cases.

It is important to treat an ulcer as soon as possible. Consult the doctor for a treatment plan. If you have an ulcer that is actively bleeding, you will most likely be admitted to the hospital for intensive care that includes endoscopy and IV ulcer medications. A blood transfusion may also be needed.

Nonsurgical Treatment

If you have a stomach ulcer caused by H. pylori, you'll need antibiotics and proton pump inhibitors (PPIs). PPIs inhibit the production of acid by stomach cells.

Your doctor might also suggest the following therapies in addition to these:

- H2 receptor antagonists (drugs that also block acid production)
- Stopping the use of all nonsteroidal anti-inflammatory drugs (NSAIDs).
- Endoscopy follow-up
- Probiotics (helpful bacteria that may have a role in destroying off H. pylori)
- Bismuth supplement

With treatment, the symptoms of an ulcer may go away quickly. And if your symptoms go away, you can continue to take the medicine your doctor has prescribed. This is especially important when dealing with H. pylori infections, as you want to make sure that all of the bacteria are gone..

When to See a Doctor

Anyone who suspects they might have a stomach ulcer should seek medical advice. Any stomach symptoms that last for more than a few days or that occur often should be evaluated and treated.

Anemia symptoms, such as fatigue and shortness of breath, may indicate a slow-bleeding ulcer. More severe bleeding is a medical emergency that can be detected by blood in the vomit or black and sticky stools.

Perforation, or a hole in the stomach, is often a life-threatening situation. The stomach wall may become infected if not treated quickly. Sudden stomach pain that worsens may be a symptom of perforation, and any symptoms of infection should be treated as soon as possible.

Home Relief For Stomach Ulcers

The following items, in addition to eating healthy foods, may help reduce the effects of H. pylori, the bacteria that causes many stomach ulcers. These supplements, however, are not meant to take the place of prescription medications or your current treatment plan. They are as follows:

- Probiotics
- Honey
- Glutaminea: type of amino acid that is found in (food sources include chicken, fish, eggs, spinach, and cabbage)

Your doctor will also have recommendations for things you should do at home to alleviate ulcer pain.

Consider discussing these natural and home remedies for ulcers with your doctor.

Risky Factors Of Developing Ulcers

Though NSAIDs are often prescribed by doctors for conditions such as arthritis or joint inflammation, they can raise the risk of developing peptic ulcers.

The following medications can increase your risk of developing gastric, duodenal, or bleeding ulcers:

- Treatments for osteoporosis, such as alendronate (Fosamax) and risedronate (Actonel)
- Anticoagulants, such as warfarin (Coumadin) or clopidogrel (Plavix)
- Selective serotonin reuptake inhibitors (SSRIs)
- Medications used in chemotherapy

Other factors that have been linked to the development of gastric and duodenal ulcers include:

- Being 70 years old or older
- Drinking alcohol
- Having a history of peptic ulcers
- Smoking
- Severe injury or physical trauma

It's a misconception that spicy foods cause or raise the risk of ulcers. However, some foods can irritate the stomach even more in certain people.

Determining Whether You Have An Ulcer

Your physician will begin by inquiring about your medical history and current symptoms. Tell your doctor when and where you are most likely to experience symptoms.

Ulcers in the stomach and duodenum may cause pain in various sections of the abdomen. Since there are so many causes of abdominal pain, a number of tests may normally be prescribed.

If your doctor suspects H. pylori as the cause of your symptoms, you can have the following tests done to confirm or rule it out:

- ✓ **A blood test is required**. You may have an H. pylori infection if you have certain infection-fighting cells in your gut.
- ✓ **A stool antigen test is performed**. A stool sample is sent to a lab for examination in this test. The test looks for certain H. pylori-related proteins in the stool.

- ✓ **A breath screening for urea.** A urea breath test entails swallowing a pill containing a specific urea formulation. Before and after swallowing the tablet, you breathe into a storage bag, and the carbon dioxide levels are measured.. When H. pylori is present, the urea in the pill is broken down into a recognizable type of carbon dioxide.

- ✓ **Esophagogastroduodenoscopy (EGD) is also performed.** Which entails passing a lighted flexible instrument with a camera on one end, known as a lens, through your mouth and down into your esophagus, stomach, and small intestine. Your doctor will check for ulcers and other abnormalities, as well as take a tissue sample (biopsy). They may even be able to diagnose certain conditions.

- ✓ **Upper gastrointestinal series.** A barium swallow or an upper GI series can be approved by your doctor. This test entails consuming a solution containing a tiny amount of liquid content that shows up clearly on an X-ray. Following that, the doctor will perform a series of X-rays to determine how the solution passes through the digestive system. This enables them to search for diseases of the esophagus, liver, and small intestine.

Methods For Treating Ulcers

The severity of your symptoms and the causes of your gastric and duodenal ulcers will determine how you are treated. To reduce the amount of acid in your stomach and protect the lining, your doctor can prescribe histamine receptor blockers (H2 blockers) or proton pump inhibitors (PPIs)..

Antibiotics, PPIs, and other medications will be prescribed by your doctor to combat H. pylori infections and promote healing. These drugs contain mucosal protective agents, which help protect the mucus lining of your stomach.

If NSAIDs triggered your peptic ulcer, you'll probably be told to cut down or stop taking them.

If the ulcer is actively bleeding, the doctor will use special instruments to stop it during the EGD procedure with the aid of an endoscope.

In the likelihood that medication or endoscopic therapy fails, your doctor can suggest surgery.. If the ulcer becomes deep enough to create a hole in the stomach or duodenum wall, it is a medical emergency, and surgery is usually needed to correct the problem.

Prognosis For Ulcers

A gastric or duodenal ulcer that goes untreated can become a serious problem, particularly if you have some medical conditions.

The most common complications of ulcers are:

- Bleeding: The stomach or small intestine is worn away by ulcers, which disrupt the blood vessels.
- Perforation: When an ulcer breaks through the stomach lining and wall, bacteria, acid, and food spill out.
- Peritonitis.
- Perforation of the abdomen causes inflammation and infection.
- Blockage.

As a result of the ulcers, scar tissue may develop, preventing food from leaving the stomach or duodenum.

If you have signs of gastric or duodenal ulcers, it's important to get properly diagnosed and treated.

Gastric ulcers can increase the risk of cancerous tumor growth in some cases. Duodenal ulcers, on the other hand, are rarely linked to cancer.

After surgery, the doctor would likely prescribe an EGD to confirm that the ulcers have healed. With time and proper medical care, most esophageal ulcers can heal.

Ways Of Preventing Ulcers

While you may not be able to fully eliminate the risk of developing an ulcer, there are steps you may take to reduce the risk and avoid it:

- If you're taking NSAIDs on a daily basis, you can cut back or turn to another drug.

- Take NSAIDs with meals or drugs to protect your stomach lining if you must take them.

- Avoid smoking because it delays healing and increases the risk of digestive cancers.

- If you've been diagnosed with H. pylori, make sure you take all of your antibiotics. If you don't finish the course, the bacteria will remain in your bloodstream.

- Increase your physical activity by taking the necessary steps. Exercise can help to stimulate the immune system and reduce inflammation in the cells.

Food Preparation And Meal Planning For Stomach Ulcers. (Both For Adults And Children)

Although there is no meal plan for everyone, these tips can help you improve your daily nutrition intake:

- Eat 4 to 6 small food daily.
- Stay hydrated — drink sufficient to hold your urine mild yellow to clear — with water, broth, tomato juice or a rehydration solution.
- Drink slowly and keep away from the use of a straw, which could motive you to ingest air, which may also reason gas.
- Prepare food in advance, and maintain your kitchen stocked with meals which you tolerate well
- Use easy cooking techniques — boil, grill, steam, poach.
- Use a food diary to record your diet and any symptoms you may experience.

How To Feed Especially When You Have Stomach Ulcers

When you have gastrointestinal inflammation flares, you may need to avoid certain foods, and other foods may help you get the right amount of nutrients, vitamins, and minerals without worsening your symptoms. Your medical team may advise you to abstain from eating and drinking, and you should avoid certain foods to identify foods that cause symptoms. This process will help you identify common foods to avoid during an outbreak. Elimination diet should only be done under the supervision of your medical team and nutritionist to ensure that you are still receiving the necessary nutrients. Some foods may cause cramps, bloating and/or diarrhea. If you have been diagnosed with stenosis, a narrowing of the intestines due to inflammation or scar tissue, or have recently had surgery, you should also avoid many trigger foods. Certain foods are easier to digest and can provide you with the necessary nutrients your body need.

Eating During Stomach Flare

When you have stomach ulcers and are in a flare attack, avoid eating foods that may cause other symptoms, and choose nutritious and nutritious foods. Watch and listen for more information about dietary advice during an outbreak.

Feeding When You Are Recovering

Even after the condition is relieved and the symptoms are reduced or disappeared, it is important to maintain a diverse and nutritious diet. Slowly introduce new food. Remember to keep the water, broth, and tomato juice and rehydration fluid. Please consult your doctor or dietitian before making any changes to your diet.

These foods can help you live healthy and hydrated:

- ✓ **Foods rich in Fiber**: Barley, cereals, oat bran, legumes, nuts and whole foods. **Protein**: lean meat, fish, eggs, nuts and tofu. Fruits and vegetables: Try to eat as much "color" as possible. If they bother you, remove the peel and seeds.

✓ **Foods rich in calcium**: kale, yogurt, kefir and milk. If you are not lactose tolerant, please choose lactose-free dairy products or use lactase digestive enzymes.

✓ **Foods containing probiotics**: yogurt, kimchi, miso, sauerkraut.

Foods don't cause stomach ulcers, but many patients find that eating certain ingredients can exacerbate the condition.

Dietary recommendations for the disease include having frequent small meals instead of large ones and avoiding carbonated beverages, hot spices and high-fiber foods.

MEAL IDEAS FOR STOMACH ULCERS

If you have stomach ulcers, which is an inflammatory disease of the large intestine, it is not always easy. Meal planning can be a difficult chore for women with stomach ulcers. Remember that Food does not cause stomach ulcers; however, many patients find that consuming certain ingredients can exacerbate this condition. Dietary prescription for the disease include: frequent small meals, avoid carbonated drinks, spicy spices and high-fiber foods.

These are some foods that may exacerbate the patient's symptoms:

- Alcohol
- caffeine
- Milk and dairy products (because many people with stomach ulcers are also lactose intolerant)
- Whole grain legumes (beans and peas)
- Fatty meats
- Dried fruits berries or anything with small seeds nuts
- Spicy and hot sauce
- Unprocessed vegetables, such as broccoli and cabbage, corn and mushrooms, may be difficult to digest.

- Food with sulfate (as a preservative)
- Acidic foods such as citrus
- All herbs and spices (in some patients instead of chopped or powdered Spices)
- Products containing sorbitol and other sugar alcohols that are used to sweeten sugar-free products

FODMAP Food

You may also have heard of something called a low FODMAP diet (here is the absurd full name: fermentable oligosaccharides, disaccharides, monosaccharides and polyols). FODMAPs are carbohydrates that are poorly absorbed in the small intestine. When they land in the colon, colonic bacteria ferment undigested sugars to produce gas. Some studies have shown that following this diet can help reduce inflammation.

High FODMAP foods include:
- Lactose foods
- Rye, wheat and barley

- Foods with fructose like apples, honey, and pears
- Foods that contain polyols, like stone fruits, mushroomsand cauliflower

Low FODMAP foods include:

- Almond and soy milk
- Cantaloupe, grapes, kiwi
- Eggs, tofu, plain lean meats
- Cucumber, potato, zucchini

Mealtime Tips

✓ **Simply prepare food**: Yes, this is simple code. Instead of frying food or immersing it in a lot of oil, choose steaming, grilling or boiling food.

✓ **Stay hydrate**: For patients with stomach ulcer, hydration is particularly important. Make sure to drink plenty of water throughout the day and choose general hydrating foods such as soups. A good way to tell you if there are enough fluids is to check the color of your urine; it should range from light yellow to clear. Darker yellow is a sign that you need to drink even more.

✓ **Choose low-fiber fruits**: Although certain fruits (such as apples, oranges, and peaches) can hardly tolerate ulcers due to their insoluble fiber content, low-fiber foods such as cantaloupe, nectar, and bananas have a milder effect on the stomach. Cooking fruits can also make them easier to digest. Fruits made into smoothies can also be eaten.

✓ **Choose vegetables wisely**: Vegetables are a key part of any diet, but when you have stomach ulcers, you should pay attention to which vegetables to eat and how to eat them. Choose non-cruciferous vegetables (usually healthy choices, but they are notorious gas-producing plants, which are exactly what you don't want during the flare) and skinless and seedless choices such as asparagus tips, potatoes and squash. Fully cooked vegetables can also help you digest them more easily.

✓ **Go for refined grains:** Foods such as white rice, white pasta, and oatmeal may be easier to digest during an outbreak. On the other hand, whole grains and whole nuts contain a lot of insoluble fiber, which can be difficult to digest.

✓ **Incorporate lean proteins:** Poultry and other meats with thin slices of lean meat, as well as fish, soybeans, eggs, and tofu, can complement the ulcer diet well and help you get the protein your body needs. This is important, especially if you have been losing weight.

✓ **Stick to "safe" food**: If you find a meal or two that you can successfully endure during an outbreak, keep that knowledge in your diary. (Hope you will know what it is, because you have been following it!) Sometimes, you already know some light meal and snack ideas that suit you can help.

PLANT-BASE-BELLY-SOOTHING RECIPES FOR OLD AND NEWLY DIAGNOSED

The food tolerance of patients with stomach ulcers is different. Elimination of certain diets can help identify problematic foods. The most common culprits are lactose, high-fat and raw fiber foods, these same foods are easily tolerated during remission. It is also important that every meal contains as many vitamins and minerals as possible, because stomach ulcers affect the absorption of nutrients during digestion. Despite these potential limitations, a healthy diet is important because his disorder can lead to nutritional deficiencies. You may need to experiment repeatedly to find out whether certain foods increase gastrointestinal discomfort, so how to avoid aggravating the ulcer while preparing healthy foods.

Try the following recipes, which do not contain dairy products, citrus, grains and other ingredients that may cause symptoms. Items you may be sensitive to are marked as optional. If any other ingredients cause you trouble, please exclude them.

Try the following recipes to make wholesome home-cooked dishes that will not worsen your symptoms.

Breakfasts Recipes

Peanut Butter-Banana Green Smoothie

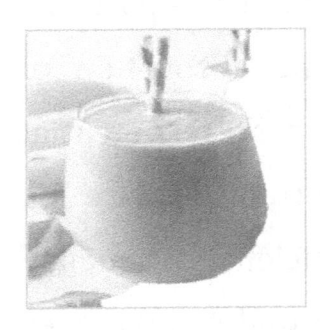

Consider using this low FODMAP milkshake for your all-in-one breakfast. stomach ulcers can destroy your ability to absorb nutrients. This smoothie can help you get the essentials you need: Spinach is a good source of iron-a mineral that is at risk of deficiency in flares. Banana helps to replace lost nutrients like potassium, which is important for electrolyte balance.

Serving Size 1

Prep and Cook Time: 5 min.

Ingredients

- 1 cup fresh spinach
- 1 medium frozen banana, sliced
- ¼ cup old-fashioned rolled oats
- ½ tsp. ground cinnamon
- 1 cup unsweetened vanilla soymilk
- 1 Tbsp. natural salted peanut butter

Nutrition Information

Per Serving: 385 Calories; 14g Fat; 2g Saturated Fat; 0mg Cholesterol; 182mg Sodium; 51g Carbohydrate; 9g Fiber; 16g Protein; 16g Sugar; 377mg Calcium; 4mg Iron; 801mg Potassium

Preparation

Mix all the ingredients in a high powder blender; blend until smooth. Served topped with strawberries (if desired).

Avocado-Egg Salad Toast

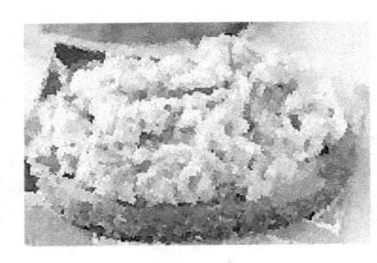

Give your eggs an extra dose to fight omega-3s. Avocados can help replenish the potassium lost due to diarrhea caused by ulcer flares. This is when you really want to choose whole wheat bread instead of white bread: it has lower fiber content and is easier to digest

Serving Size: 4

Prep and Cook Time: 10 min.

Ingredients

- 1 large ripe avocado
- ¼ tsp. black pepper
- 4 hard-boiled eggs, diced
- 1 Tbsp. fresh lemon juice
- ½ tsp. kosher salt
- 4 slices white sourdough bread, toasted
- 1 Tbsp. chopped fresh parsley, plus more for garnish

Nutrition Information

Per serving: 328 Calories; 14g Fat; 3g Saturated Fat; 186mg Cholesterol; 700mg Sodium; 38g Carbohydrate; 5g Fiber; 14g Protein; 4g Sugar; 66mg Calcium; 4mg Iron; 397mg Potassium

Preparation

1. Cut the avocado in half and then remove the core. Remove the flesh from the skin and put it in a bowl. Mash thoroughly using a fork. Add the diced eggs, lemon juice, parsley, salt and pepper.

2. Divide mixture equally onto each slice of toasted bread. Garnish with additional parsley, if desired.

Ginger Elixir

This is an easy to make Ayurvedic Digestive Drink, best to have during fall and winter season. Ginger acts wonders to fire up our digestive system.

Ingredients

- 1/2 lime/lemon juice
- 1 cup water
- 1 teaspoon pure maple syrup
- 1-2 inch grated fresh ginger
- A pinch of Himalayan salt

- 1/4 teaspoon crushed black pepper

Preparation

Blend all ingredients in a blender until smooth

For the sweetener, you could even use turbinado sugar or honey (if not a strict vegan). The key is to not to make this drink too sweet, you need to taste the pungency of ginger and heat of the black pepper when you drink this. This is what aids in better digestion.

Whole-Grain Morning Glory Muffins

These healthy breakfast treats have walnuts, which may offer protection against stomach ulcers. Walnuts contain omega-3 fatty acids, eating them will offer preventative benefits in ulcer patients, resulting less damage from inflammation leading up to flare, plus faster healing after.

Serving Size: 12

Prep and Cook Time: 1 hr.

Ingredients

- 3 large eggs
- ½ cup raisins
- 2 cups white whole-wheat flour
- 2 tsp. baking soda
- 2 tsp. ground cinnamon
- 1 tsp. ground cardamom
- 1 tsp. ground ginger
- Cooking spray
- ¼ tsp. kosher salt
- ¾ cup unsweetened applesauce
- ½ cup vegetable oil
- ½ cup pure maple syrup
- 2 tsp. vanilla extract
- ½ cup chopped walnuts
- 1 cup finely grated carrots

Nutrition Information

Per Serving: 260 Calories; 15g Fat; 2g Saturated Fat; 45mg Cholesterol; 277mg Sodium; 30g Carbohydrate; 3g Fiber; 5g Protein; 14g Sugar; 37mg Calcium; 1mg Iron; 215mg Potassium

Preparation

1. Preheat your oven to 350°F. Grease your 12 muffin cups, or arrange with paper liners.

2. In a sizeable bowl, combine together flour, baking soda, cinnamon, cardamom, ginger, and salt. Set aside.

3. In a separate bowl, whisk eggs, applesauce, oil, maple syrup, and vanilla until combined. Stir in carrots.

4. Pour wet ingredients into dry ingredients; stir until just well mixed. Fold in raisins and walnuts.

5. Divide the batter equally into your prepared muffin tins. Bake in preheated oven for 20 minutes, or until a toothpick inserted in the center of a muffin comes out mostly clean.

6. Allow to cool for 15 minutes before removing from muffin tin and transfer to a wire rack to cool completely, and then serve. Store the remaining in an air-tight container or refrigerate

Fluffy Blueberry Oatmeal Pancakes

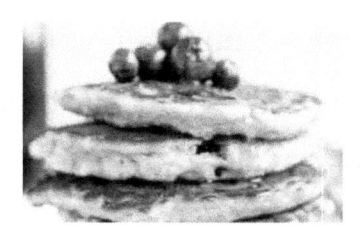

Whole wheat flour and oatmeal can provide a double dose of whole wheat food, which can enhance the body's anti-inflammatory compounds.

Serving Size: 3

Prep and Cook Time: 30 min.

Ingredients

- ½ cup quick-cooking oats
- ¾ cup white whole-wheat flour
- 1 tsp. baking powder
- Cooking spray
- ½ tsp. ground cinnamon
- ¼ tsp. salt
- 1 large egg, whisked
- 4 Tbsp. pure maple syrup, divided
- 1 Tbsp. vegetable oil
- ½ tsp. vanilla extract
- 2 Tbsp. creamy almond butter

- ¾ cup unsweetened cashew milk (or your non-dairy milk of choice) ⬚ ½ cup frozen wild blueberries, thawed, plus more for garnish

Nutrition Information

Per serving: 389 Calories; 15g Fat; 2g Saturated Fat; 62mg Cholesterol; 453mg Sodium; 54g Carbohydrate; 7g Fiber; 10g Protein; 18g Sugar; 166mg Calcium; 3mg Iron; 226mg Potassium

Preparation

1. Mix the oats and cashew milk in a medium bowl; allow for few minutes to coat.

2. Afterwards, combine flour, baking powder, cinnamon, and salt in a large bowl; stir with a whisk. Keep aside.

3. Add 1 Tbsp. of the maple syrup, oil, egg and vanilla to oat mixture; stir to mix well. Pour in the oat mixture into flour mixture; stir until just well mixed. Fold in blueberries.

4. Heat a greased nonstick skillet or griddle over medium heat. As the pan heats, mix the remaining 3 Tbsp. maple syrup and almond butter in a small bowl. Add 1 Tbsp. hot water and stir using a whisk until smooth. Keep aside.

5. Place a scant ¼ cup of pancake batter per pancake onto hot griddle. Bake until tops are covered with bubbles and edges look dry and cooked, about 3 minutes. Flip and cook 1 to 2 minutes on the other side.

6. Serve with almond butter sauce and additional blueberries, if needed.

Southwestern Sweet Potato and Egg Hash

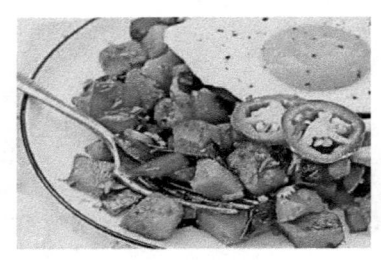

This antioxidant-rich breakfast will start the day! Breakfast hash is a great way to increase vegetable intake, which is one of the pillars of the Mediterranean diet. This is a double vitamin A that combines sweet potato and red bell pepper, which many ulcers patients lack.

Serving Size: 2

Prep and Cook Time: 25 min.

Ingredients

- 2 large eggs
- 2 ½ Tbsp. extra-virgin olive oil, divided
- ¾ cup chopped red bell pepper
- ¼ tsp. ground cumin
- ¼ cup finely chopped red onion
- ½ tsp. chili powder
- ½ tsp. kosher salt, divided

- 4 Tbsp. prepared salsa
- ½ ripe avocado, well sliced
- Fresh cilantro for garnish (optional)
- 2 cups peeled and cubed sweet potato (about ½-in. each)

Nutrition Information

Per serving: 458 Calories; 29g Fat; 5g Saturated Fat; 185mg Cholesterol; 746mg Sodium; 35g Carbohydrate; 9g Fiber; 10g Protein; 10g Sugar; 84mg Calcium; 2mg Iron; 960mg Potassium

Preparation

1. Heat 1 tbsp. oil in a large skillet over medium. Add sweet potato; cook for 5 minutes, until lightly golden. Add 3 Tbsp. water, cover, and cook until tender, stirring occasionally for about 7 minutes.

2. Add 1 Tbsp. oil, onion and bell pepper to pan with potatoes. Cook uncovered, for about 5 minutes until vegetables are tender. Season with ¼ tsp. of the salt, chili powder and cumin; divide mixture between two bowls.

3. Add remaining ½ tsp. oil to pan. Crack eggs into pan; cook for 3 to 4 minutes, or until whites are set. Season with remaining ¼ tsp. salt.

4. Place an egg on top of each potato mixture. Top each with 2 Tbsp. salsa, sliced avocado, and cilantro for garnish. Serve.

Orange-Scented Golden Overnight Oats

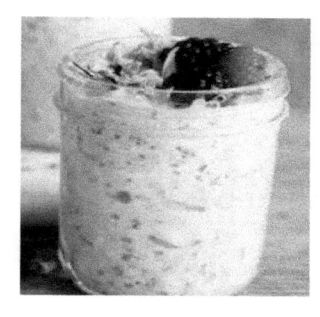

Put these oats in the refrigerator before going to bed and wake up to a delicious breakfast! The color of this dish comes from turmeric, which contains anti-inflammatory compounds, which may be beneficial for the treatment of stomach ulcers. To get a double anti-inflammatory effect, add some berries, such as raspberries or blueberries, to the oatmeal.

Serving Size: 2

Prep and Cook Time: 6 hr. 5 min.

<u>Ingredients</u>

- 2 Tbsp. pure maple syrup
- 1 cup old-fashioned rolled oats
- 1 ¼ cup unsweetened vanilla soymilk
- 1 tsp. orange zest
- ¼ tsp. kosher salt

- ¾ tsp. ground turmeric
- ¼ tsp. ground cinnamon

Optional topping

- Fresh raspberries and/or blueberries

Nutrition Information

Per serving: 261 Calories; 6g Fat; 1g Saturated Fat; 0mg Cholesterol; 296mg Sodium; 43g Carbohydrate; 6g Fiber; 9g Protein; 14g Sugar; 241mg Calcium; 3mg Iron; 373mg Potassium

Preparation

Combine the all ingredients (except the berries if using) in a container or Mason jar; stir well. Cover and refrigerate for 6 hours, or overnight. Garnish with fresh berries, if needed.

Smoked-Salmon Breakfast Bake

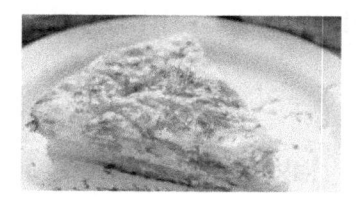

Salmon and eggs are good sources of vitamin D for bone strengthening, and many people with ulcers lack vitamin D. Studies prove that this fat-soluble vitamin can also help relieve Inflammation of the guts.

Serving Size: 6

Prep and Cook Time: 50 min.

<u>Ingredients</u>

- ¼ tsp. salt
- 10 large eggs
- 1 tsp. Dijon mustard
- ¼ tsp. black pepper
- 2 Tbsp. extra-virgin olive oil
- 2 oz. goat cheese, well crumbled

- ¼ cup finely chopped red onion
- 2 Tbsp. minced fresh chives, divided
- 12 oz. russet potatoes, peeled and cut into ½ in. cubes
- 6 oz. hot-smoked salmon, flaked (find it near the fresh-fish counter)

Nutrition Information

Per serving: 295 Calories; 18g Fat; 6g Saturated Fat; 338mg Cholesterol; 518mg Sodium; 12g Carbohydrate; 1g Fiber; 21g Protein; 1g Sugar; 85mg Calcium; 2mg Iron; 505mg Potassium

Preparation

1. Preheat oven to 350°F. Put 1 Tbsp. chives, eggs, mustard, salt, and pepper in a sizable bowl; whisk to well combine. Keep aside.

2. Heat oil in a 10-inch oven-safe skillet over medium temperature. Add the potatoes, stir well to coat, arrange in a single layer. Cover and cook until potatoes are almost done, about 8 minutes, stirring occasionally. Add red onion; cook for additional 3 minutes, until softened.

3. Place the salmon equally over potato mixture in pan. Pour egg mixture over salmon and potatoes. Drizzle cheese on top, and place pan to preheated oven. Bake egg for 25 minutes, or until mixture is set.

4. Garnish with remaining 1 Tbsp. chives. Allow to cool for 5 minutes before cutting into 6 slices. Serve.

Spinach and Red-Pepper Muffin-Tin Frittatas

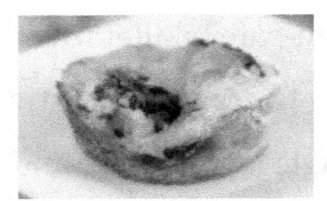

Eggs are an important source of protein and are usually well tolerated during attacks of stomach ulcers. For extra anti-inflammatory ability, choose a brand that has fortified omega-3 fatty acids. Eat a batch of these low FODMAP eggs throughout the week.

Serving Size: 6

Prep and Cook Time: 40 min.

Ingredients

- 12 large eggs
- Cooking spray
- 1 tsp. kosher salt
- 4 oz. fresh spinach
- 2 tsp. olive oil
- ½ tsp. black pepper
- frozen shredded hash browns
- 1 red bell pepper, well chopped
- Fresh avocado slices for serving (optional)

- 12 oz. refrigerated unseasoned shredded hash brown potatoes (or use thawed

Nutrition Information

Per serving: 217 calories; 11g fat; 3g saturated fat; 372mg cholesterol; 514mg sodium; 14g carbohydrate; 2g fiber; 15g protein; 1g sugar; 75mg calcium; 2mg iron; 272mg potassium

Preparation

1. Preheat your oven to 400°F. Divide potatoes equally into 12 greased muffin cups; press into bottoms and slightly up sides. Bake for 15 minutes, or until lightly golden.

2. Afterwards, heat oil in a sizeable skillet over medium temperature. Add bell pepper, and cook until softened, about 5 to 6 minutes. Add spinach, and cook until wilted, stirring frequently, about 1 minute. Spread the

vegetable mixture equally in each muffin tin over cooked potatoes.

3. Whisk the eggs, add salt, and pepper in a large bowl, and pour equally into each muffin cup. Place back in the oven and heat until eggs are just set, about 10 to 12 minutes. Allow to cool for 5 minutes before removing from pan.

4. Serve with sliced avocado, if desired. Refrigerate leftovers in an airtight bag; reheat in a microwave or toaster oven.

Lunches Recipes

Tahini-Caesar Chicken Pitas

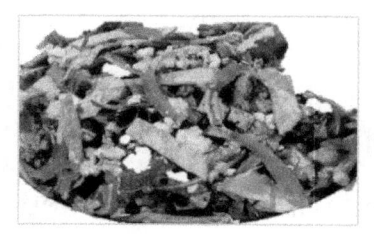

Since many ulcer patients suffer from dairy intolerance, this Caesar seasoning is made with tahini. Tahini is a sesame paste rich in antioxidants. Choosing whole-wheat pita bread can get many benefits of added fiber, such as slower digestion and added micronutrients.

Serving Size: 4

Prep and Cook Time: 20 min.

<u>Ingredients</u>

- ¾ tsp. kosher salt, divided
- ½ tsp. paprika
- ¾ tsp. black pepper, divided
- ½ tsp. dried oregano
- 1 Tbsp. fresh lemon juice
- Cooking spray
- ⅓ cup thinly sliced red onion
- 3 Tbsp. tahini (sesame seed paste)

- 1 lb. boneless, skinless chicken breasts
- 1 tsp. finely chopped capers
- 1 tsp. Dijon mustard
- ½ tsp. granulated garlic or garlic powder
- 1 cup canned chickpeas, rinsed and drained
- 4 cups chopped romaine lettuce
- 4 (3-oz.) whole-grain pita pockets, sliced in half

Nutrition Information

Per serving: 506 Calories; 12g Fat; 2g Saturated Fat; 83mg Cholesterol; 1082mg Sodium; 63g Carbohydrate; 10g Fiber; 40g Protein; 4g Sugar; 81mg Calcium; 5mg Iron; 826mg Potassium

Preparation

1. Season the chicken wholly with ½ tsp. salt, ½ tsp. black pepper, oregano, and paprika.

2. Heat a grill pan over medium-high temperature. Use cooking spray to coat pan and chicken breasts. Put the chicken; cook for 5 minutes on each side or until done. Remove cooked chicken from pan; let cool for 5 minutes. Slice chicken thinly across the grain.

3. Afterwards, prepare Tahini-Caesar dressing by combining tahini, lemon juice, capers, mustard, garlic, and remaining ¼ tsp. each salt and black pepper. Slowly whisk in up to 3 Tbsp. warm water and mixed until smooth.

4. Add lettuce, red onion, and chickpeas in a sizeable bowl; toss with half of Tahini-Caesar dressing. Divide the lettuce mixture and chicken equally among pita halves; sprinkle on each stuffed pita with remaining Tahini Caesar dressing.

Butternut Squash Soup with Lemongrass

Low FODMAP soup can help the belly heal. When ulcers attack, peeled, cooked and mixed vegetables are easy to digest. This soothing soup also provides anti-inflammatory compounds through turmeric and ginger.

Serving Size: 4

Prep and Cook Time: 1 hr.

<u>Ingredients</u>

- ½ tsp. kosher salt
- ½ tsp. ground turmeric
- 1 Tbsp. minced fresh ginger
- 2 Tbsp. extra-virgin olive oil
- 4 cups lower-sodium vegetable broth
- 4 cups peeled and cubed butternut squash
- Microgreens or fresh basil for garnish (optional)

- 2 ½ cups chopped carrots (about 3 large carrots)
- 1 Tbsp. lemongrass paste (find it in tubes near the fresh-herb case)
- ½ cup plus 4 tsp. coconut-milk yogurt, divided (or use the same amount canned coconut milk)

Nutrition Information

Per Serving: 226 Calories; 9g Fat; 2g Saturated Fat; 3mg Cholesterol; 556mg Sodium; 32g Carbohydrate; 6g Fiber; 5g Protein; 12g Sugar; 143mg Calcium; 2mg Iron; 753mg Potassium

<u>Preparation</u>

1. Preheat oil in a Dutch oven or sizeable stockpot over medium heat. Add squash and carrots; cook and stir occasionally for 5 minutes, until lightly golden. Add ginger, lemongrass paste, turmeric, and salt; cook for 2 minutes, until aromatic.

2. Add broth and increase heat to high. Allow mixture to boil, and then reduce heat to medium-low, cover and cook, for 25 minutes, or until vegetables are tender.

3. Gently pour the mixture into the blender; add a cup of yogurt. Remove the central part of the blender cover (so that the steam can escape); fix the cover on the blender. Put a clean towel on the opening of the lid. Processing until smooth.

4. Divide soup equally into 6 serving plates. Swirl 1 tsp. yogurt into each serving, and garnish with fresh basil or micro greens, if needed.
5.

Fried Rice with Miso-Turmeric Vinaigrette

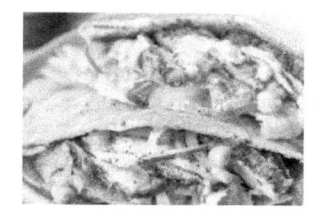

White rice has lower fiber content than brown, so when your ulcer symptoms occur, white rice is easier to digest. The dressing provides anti-inflammatory compounds of turmeric and ginger, as well as probiotics that taste miso, to help restore intestinal bacteria.

Serving Size: 4

Prep and Cook Time: 20 min.

Ingredients

- 2 Tbsp. unseasoned rice vinegar
- 1 cup matchstick carrots
- 2 Tbsp. sesame oil (not toasted)
- 2 Tbsp. vegetable oil
- 2 tsp. white miso paste
- ½ tsp. freshly grated ginger
- 3 large eggs, whisked
- ¼ tsp. ground turmeric
- 2 cups roughly chopped baby bok choy

- 2 ½ cups cooked white rice
- 2 Tbsp. lower-sodium soy sauce
- 2 Tbsp. chopped fresh basil

Nutrition Information

Per serving: 322 Calories; 18g Fat; 3g Saturated Fat; 140mg Cholesterol; 443mg Sodium; 32g Carbohydrate; 1g Fiber; 9g Protein; 2g Sugar; 68mg Calcium; 2mg Iron; 92mg Potassium

Preparation

1. Prepare sauce by mixing the vinegar, sesame oil, miso, ginger, and turmeric in a small container; stir with a whisk. Set aside.

2. Heat vegetable oil in a sizeable skillet over medium-high temperature. Add bok choy and carrots; cook for 5 minutes, stirring occasionally, until tender. Pour in the rice and soy sauce, and press rice down evenly in the

skillet. Cook all through, until bottom of rice begins to crisp, about 3 minutes. Toss to combine.

3. Push the rice and vegetables to all sides, opening a large opening in the center of the pot. Pour in the eggs and beat them thoroughly, until the eggs are messed up, about 1 to 2 minutes. Mix the egg and rice mixture well, then stir in the basil.

4. Distribute fried rice equally between each of 4 serving plates. Sprinkle Miso Turmeric Vinaigrette on top.

Greek Chicken Pasta Salad

This salad is a bowl of Med. diet. This fresh pasta salad is enough for your dinner! Patients with stomach ulcers who adhere to a Mediterranean diet rich in anti-inflammatory foods may have fewer attacks. Since ingredients such as olive oil and olives provide antioxidant polyphenol plus lean protein and vegetables.

Serving Size: 6

Prep and Cook Time: 30 min.

Ingredients

- 1 lb. boneless, skinless chicken breasts
- ½ tsp. paprika
- 1 tsp. kosher salt, divided
- ½ tsp. black pepper
- Cooking spray
- 12 oz. dry fusilli or rotini pasta
- 2 tsp. minced fresh garlic
- 2 tsp. Dijon mustard
- 4 cups fresh baby spinach
- 2 tbsp. red wine vinegar

- ¼ cup extra-virgin olive oil
- 1-pint cherry tomatoes, halved
- 1 (14-oz.) can artichoke hearts, drained
- 1 tbsp. finely chopped fresh oregano
- 1 (2.25-oz.) can sliced black olives, drained
- ½ cup crumbled feta cheese (optional)

Nutrition Information

Per serving: 465 Calories; 14g Fat; 2g Saturated Fat; 55mg Cholesterol; 913mg Sodium; 54g Carbohydrate; 5g Fiber; 28g Protein; 4g Sugar; 59mg Calcium; 4mg Iron; 462mg Potassium

Preparation

1. Season the chicken evenly with a teaspoon of salt, black pepper and chili powder. Heat the grill pan over medium high heat.

2. Coat the pan and chicken breast with cooking spray. Add chicken; cook for 5 minutes on each

side or until cooked through. Remove the chicken from the pan; let it cool for 5 minutes. Cut the chicken into small pieces.

3. Afterwards, according to the package instructions, cook the pasta in salty water and cook until it's cooked. Drain the water and rinse with cold water.

4. Meanwhile, mix the garlic, mustard, red wine vinegar, oregano and remaining ½ tsp. salt in a bowl; mix with a whisk. Gradually stream in olive oil, whisking often, until combined.

5. Then, put the tomatoes, spinach, artichoke hearts and black olives into the pasta bowl; stir well. Add chicken, feta and seasoning; toss it up.

Sweet Potato and Lentil Soup

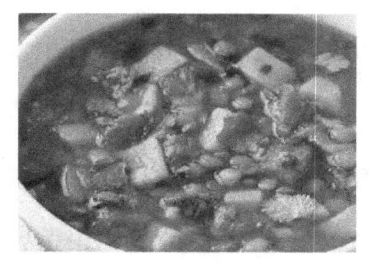

When inflammation is relieved, beans (such as lentils) can provide you with the ideal fiber and protein dosage. You will also get β-carotene (the precursor of vitamin A) from sweet potatoes.

Serving Size: 6

Prep and Cook Time: 50 min.

Ingredients

- 2 Tbsp. extra-virgin olive oil
- 3 garlic cloves
- 1 cup chopped yellow onion
- 2 Tbsp. tomato paste
- 2 tsp. garam masala
- 1 tsp. kosher salt
- 2 tsp. ground cumin

- 4 cups lower-sodium vegetable broth
- 2 cups water
- 1 (14.5-oz.) can fire-roasted tomatoes
- 1 large sweet potato, peeled and cut into ½-in. pieces (about 2 cups)
- 1 cup uncooked brown lentils
- 1 bunch Lacinato kale, stemmed and roughly chopped ▢ Fresh parsley for garnish (optional)

Nutrition Information

Per serving: 254 Calories; 6g Fat; 1g Saturated Fat; 0mg Cholesterol; 652mg Sodium; 21g Carbohydrate; 4g Fiber; 12g Protein; 8g Sugar; 125mg Calcium; 6mg Iron; 612mg Potassium

Preparation

1. Heat the oil over medium heat in a sizeable saucepan or Dutch oven. Add onions; cook for 5 minutes, until tender. Add garlic, tomato paste, cumin and garam masala; cook for 2 minutes,

stirring occasionally. Add sweet potatoes; stir and cook for 5 minutes. Add the lentils.

2. Add broth, water, salt and tomatoes; allow the mixture to boil. Reduce the heat, simmer on low heat, and cover until the lentils are cooked and the sweet potatoes are tender, about 30 to 35 minutes. Pour in the kale and stir and cook until the kale is wilted for about 2 minutes.

3. Divide equally into 6 serving. If needed, you can garnish with fresh parsley.

Quinoa Taco Salads with Chili-Lime Vinaigrette

You will never miss the meat in this vegan vegetable taco salad. Some studies have pointed out that high-fat red meat may cause symptoms of stomach ulcers. Therefore, this taco salad replaces ground beef (which is high in saturated fat). It uses zesty-spicy quinoa, which is a thin source of plant-based protein.

Serving Size: 4

Prep and Cook Time: 45 min.

Ingredients

- 1 cup lower-sodium vegetable broth
- 2 tsp. prepared taco seasoning
- 1 tsp. lime zest, plus 2 Tbsp. fresh lime juice (separate)
- ½ tsp. chili powder
- ½ cup dry quinoa, well rinsed
- ½ tsp. kosher salt, divided
- 1 ½ tsp. pure maple syrup
- ¼ cup extra-virgin olive oil
- 8 cups chopped romaine lettuce
- 1 ripe avocado, well sliced
- 1 cup frozen fire-roasted corn, thawed
- 1-pint cherry tomatoes, halved
- 1 (15-oz.) can black beans, well rinsed and drained

- ⅓ cup thinly sliced red onion

Nutrition Information

Per serving: 374 Calories; 23g Fat; 3g Saturated Fat; 0mg Cholesterol; 704mg Sodium; 37g Carbohydrate; 12g Fiber; 9g Protein; 6g Sugar; 92mg Calcium; 3mg Iron; 768mg Potassium

Preparation

1. Combine the quinoa, broth, and taco seasoning in a small pot over medium high heat; bring to a boil. Cover the lid, reduce the heat to low-medium level, and simmer until the soup is absorbed, about 15 minutes.

2. Remove from the heat; stand up, cover the pot, let it sit for 15 minutes, then fluff it with a fork. Put it in a bowl and transfer to the refrigerator to cool.

3. While waiting, mix the lime zest and juice, chili powder, ¼ tsp. salt, and maple syrup in a small bowl; stir well using whisk. Carefully stream in oil, whisking continuously, until combined.
4. Place lettuce, black beans, corn, onions, tomatoes and the remaining teaspoons of salt in a large bowl; toss it up. Distribute equally among four bowls. Remove the quinoa from the refrigerator and spoon equally on the salad. Drizzle chili lime balsamic vinegar on top and sprinkle sliced avocado on each salad.

Tuna Niçoise Grain Bowl

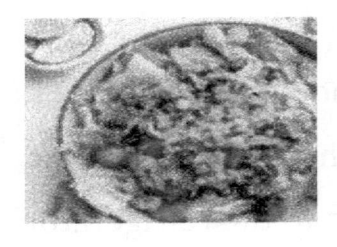

During the remission period, patients with stomach ulcers are encouraged to follow the Mediterranean diet, focusing on fish rich in omega 3, such as salmon and tuna, as well as whole grains, olive oil and fresh produce. This full bowl has everything and more.

Serving Size: 4

Prep and Cook Time: 40 min.

<u>Ingredients</u>

- 2 tsp. honey
- 1 cup dry farro, rinsed
- ½ tsp. kosher salt, divided
- 12 oz. small red or fingerling potatoes
- 6 oz. haricots verts (French green beans)
- 2 Tbsp. fresh lemon juice
- 2 tsp. chopped fresh oregano or ¾ tsp. dried
- 1 tsp. Dijon mustard
- ¼ tsp. black pepper
- ¼ cup extra-virgin olive oil
- 2 oz. black or green olives, sliced
- 1 cup halved cherry tomatoes
- 2 (5-oz.) cans tuna, drained and flaked
- 2 soft-boiled eggs, halved (optional)

Nutrition Information

Per serving: 489 Calories; 19g Fat; 3g Saturated Fat; 30mg Cholesterol; 688mg Sodium; 30mg Carbohydrate; 6g Fiber; 26g Protein; 7g Sugar; 81mg Calcium; 3mg Iron; 814mg Potassium

Preparation

1. Place farro in a small saucepan; add ¼ tsp. salt and 3 cups water. Allow to boil; lower the heat to medium-low, and simmer, with the lid covered, for 30 minutes. Drain any excess liquid.

2. Meanwhile, Place the potatoes in a separate large pot; add water to cover 2 inches. Bring to a high boil; reduce to medium-low level, then cook for 15 minutes. Add the haricots; cook for another 6 minutes. Drain and rinse the potatoes

and haricots. Cut the potatoes into halves or quarters according to their size. Set aside.

3. Place the lemon juice, oregano, honey, mustard, remaining salt and black pepper in a small bowl; stir to combine. Gradually infuse olive oil, stirring constantly until smooth.

4. Divide the cooked farro, potatoes, haricots, tomatoes, tuna and olives evenly into four bowls. Add half an egg to each bowl, then drizzle the dressing on top.

Lemony Orzo Salad with Flaked Salmon

Simple pasta with salmon rich in omega can soothe an angry belly. It looks a bit like rice, but orzo is actually a short-cut white pasta that has low fiber content and is easy in the belly of ulcers patients. Salmon provides omega-3 fatty acids EPA and DHA, which can help relieve systemic inflammation.

Serving Size: 4

Prep and Cook Time: 45 min.

Ingredients

- 1 cup uncooked orzo
- 2 cups lower-sodium vegetable broth
- ½ tsp. kosher salt, divided
- ¼ tsp. black pepper
- 2 cups fresh baby spinach
- 1 Tbsp. fresh lemon juice
- 2 (6-oz.) center-cut salmon fillets
- ⅓ cup sun-dried tomatoes packed in oil, plus 2 Tbsp. oil from jar, divided
- 2 Tbsp. fresh parsley leaves

Nutrition Information

Per serving: 374 Calories; 14g Fat; 2g Saturated Fat; 47mg Cholesterol; 395mg Sodium; 37g

Carbohydrate; 3g Fiber; 23g Protein; 3g Sugar; 55mg Calcium; 2mg Iron; 571mg Potassium

Preparation

1. Heat 1 tablespoon the sun-dried tomato oil medium -sized pot, over high heat. Add orzo; cook for 2 minutes, stirring often. Add broth and teaspoon salt; allow to boil. Cover the pot, reduce the heat, and simmer for 10 to 12 minutes, or until the broth is absorbed.

2. Remove the pan from the heat; leave covered for 5 minutes. Stir in spinach, sun-dried tomatoes and lemon juice (spinach will wilt quickly).
3. At the same time, preheat the broiler with an oven rack 6 inches from the heat. Brush salmon with 1 tablespoon of sun-dried tomato oil and season with the remaining teaspoon salt and

black pepper. Place the fillets (face down) on a foil-lined baking sheet. Broil to your desire, for 8 to 10 minutes. Use a metal spatula to remove the fillets from the foil.

4. Take away the salmon skin; use a fork to gradually pull the flesh into large flakes; toss with orzo. Divide orzo salad evenly among 4 plates; serve with fresh parsley.

Zucchini Noodles

It is smart to avoid eating high-fiber vegetables during flares, and cooked zucchini noodles are an excellent alternative for low residues. (By the way, low residue means low fiber.) The tofu here is an important source of calcium, which is especially important for ulcers patients on steroids.

Serving Size: 4

Prep and Cook Time: 20 min.

Ingredients

- 3 Tbsp. natural creamy peanut butter
- Juice of 1 lime
- 2 Tbsp. lower-sodium soy sauce
- 1 ½ tsp. freshly grated ginger
- 2 tsp. pure maple syrup
- 1 red bell pepper, thinly sliced
- 2 Tbsp. extra-virgin olive oil, divided
- 1 ½ cups matchstick carrots
- 1 (14-oz.) block extra-firm tofu, drained, patted dry, and cut into 1-in.
- cubes
- ½ tsp. kosher salt, divided
- 4 medium zucchinis, trimmed and spiralized into thin noodles

Nutrition Information

Per serving: 311 Calories; 19g Fat; 3g Saturated Fat; 0mg Cholesterol; 591mg Sodium; 20g Carbohydrate;

5g Fiber; 17g Protein; 11g Sugar; 126mg Calcium; 3mg Iron; 661mg Potassium

Preparation

1. In a small bowl, mix together peanut butter, soy sauce, ginger, lime juice and maple syrup and mix well.

2. Heat 1 tablespoon oil in a medium nonstick pan. Add tofu; cook for 8 to 10 minutes, or until the tofu is golden and crisp, stirring once a while. Season the tofu with a small ¼ teaspoon salt; transfer to a plate.

3. Add the remaining 1 tablespoon oil into the pan. Boil the carrots and bell peppers until tender, about 5 to 6 minutes, stirring occasionally. Season with the remaining ¼ teaspoon salt.

4. Put the zucchini noodles in the pot; cook for 2 to 3 minutes, turning frequently to heat, but not fully cooked. Add the tofu and half of the peanut butter to the frying pan. Toss to combine.

5. Distribute the zucchini noodle mixture evenly on 4 plates. Drizzle the remaining peanut sauce on top.

Dinners Recipes

Seared Scallops with Avocado-Citrus Salsa

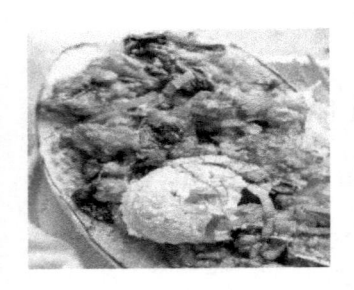

Fruits like avocado and orange are low in roughage and easier to digest when stomach ulcers symptoms are flaring up. They're also rich in vitamin C, which can enhance iron absorption (especially important if your ulcer is contributing to anemia).

Serving Size: 4

Prep and Cook Time: 30 min.

Ingredients

- ¾ cup dry quinoa, rinsed
- 1 lb. sea scallops, patted dry
- 2 cups lower-sodium vegetable broth ⏤ 2 Tbsp. extra-virgin olive oil
- 1 cup diced avocado (from 1 avocado)
- ¾ tsp. kosher salt, divided
- ½ tsp. black pepper, divided
- 2 Tbsp. chopped fresh parsley
- ¾ cup peeled and diced orange segments
- ¼ cup finely chopped red bell pepper

- 1 tsp. orange zest, plus 2 Tbsp. fresh orange juice

Nutrition Information

Per serving: 352 Calories; 15g Fat; 2g Saturated Fat; 27mg Cholesterol; 880mg Sodium; 35g Carbohydrate; 7g Fiber; 19g Protein; 6g Sugar; 58mg Calcium; 3mg Iron; 702mg Potassium

Preparation

1. In a small pan, mix the quinoa and broth and bring it to a boil. Reduce the heat to minimum, cover and simmer for about 15 minutes, until most of the broth is absorbed. Fluff quinoa using a fork and cover to keep warm.

2. Meanwhile, heat 1 Tbsp. oil in a sizeable skillet over medium-high. Drizzle scallops with ½ tsp. salt and ¼ tsp. black pepper. Add scallops to pan; cook 2 minutes. Flip and cook for 2

additional minutes or until the degree of doneness is achieved. Remove the scallops from pan and keep warm.

3. Mix the orange, avocado, segments, bell pepper, orange zest and juice, remaining 1 Tbsp. oil, ¼ tsp. salt, and ¼ tsp. black pepper in a bowl; slowly mix them up to combine.

4. Serve the quinoa and scallops equally between four serving plates. Top with Avocado-Citrus Salsa, and garnish with fresh parsley.

Spaghetti Squash Lasagna Boats with Almond Ricotta

When you have stomach ulcers, fatty ground beef and milk can worsen the symptoms. This recipe uses lean ground turkey breast and faux-ricotta cheese made of blanched almonds as an alternative.

Serving Size: 4

Prep and Cook Time: 1 hr.

<u>Ingredients</u>

- 2 medium spaghetti squashes
- 1 lb. ground turkey breast
- ⅓ cup warm water
- 2 cups fresh baby spinach
- ¾ tsp. kosher salt, divided
- 1 (15-oz.) can crushed tomatoes
- 1 tsp. nutritional yeast
- ¾ cup blanched almonds
- 2 Tbsp. extra-virgin olive oil, divided
- 2 tsp. fresh lemon juice
- 4 Tbsp. fresh chopped basil leaves, divided

Nutrition Information

Per serving: 456 Calories; 23g Fat; 3g Saturated Fat; 55mg Cholesterol; 709mg Sodium; 30g Carbohydrate; 9g Fiber; 37g Protein; 12g Sugar; 181mg Calcium; 5mg Iron; 782mg Potassium

Preparation

1. Preheat the oven to 400°F. Cut the squashes, lengthwise, in half and extract the seeds. Rub the flesh with 1 Tbsp. of oil, and position on a rimmed baking sheet, cut side down. Bake for 40 minutes, or until the flesh is soft.

2. After that, heat the remaining 1 Tbsp. oil in a sizeable skillet over medium heat. Add the turkey; cook for 6 to 7 minutes, or until fully cooked, breaking the meat into small pieces. Stir in the spinach; cook, until wilted, for 2 minutes. Season with ½ tsp. salt.

3. Pour in tomatoes and 2 Tbsp. of basil; lower the heat. Cover to keep it warm.

4. Combine the lemon juice, almonds, nutritional yeast, water, and the remaining 1/4 tsp. salt in a high-power food processor or blender. Blend until perfectly smooth.

5. Remove the spaghetti squash from the oven and shred flesh (like strands) on the spaghetti using a fork.

6. Place on each squash half with the turkey mixture. Top with 2 Tbsp. Almond Ricotta. Serve evenly with remaining 2 Tbsp. basil.

Sheet-Pan Salmon Romesco with Green Beans & Crushed Potatoes

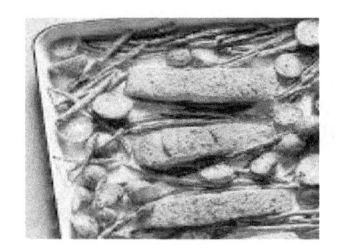

It takes only 15 minutes to prepare this easy-to-digest meal. Steer clear of high-fibre vegetables during a flare, which may worsen an already-irritated colon. Better alternatives include cooked green beans and potatoes that are naturally poor in FODMAPs. Discomfort or bloating is the last thing you need when you have stomach ulcers.

Serving Size: 4

Prep and Cook Time: 45 min.

<u>Ingredients</u>
- 12 oz. baby yellow potatoes
- 1 lb. skin-on salmon, sliced into 4 fillets
- ¼ cup walnuts
- 1 tsp. kosher salt, divided
- ¾ tsp. black pepper, divided
- ¼ tsp. paprika
- 8 oz. haricots verts (French green beans)
- ¾ cup jarred roasted red peppers, drained
- 2 Tbsp. plus 2 tsp. extra-virgin olive oil, divided
- 2 tsp. fresh lemon juice
- Fresh parsley for garnish (optional)

Nutrition Information

Per serving: 376 Calories; 21g Fat; 3g Saturated Fat; 62mg Cholesterol; 781mg Sodium; 23g Carbohydrate; 4g Fiber; 26g Protein; 4g Sugar; 105mg Calcium; 3mg Iron; 715mg Potassium

Preparation

1. Preheat the oven to 425°F. Put the potatoes in a small saucepan; containing water, boil and simmer for 12 minutes, or until almost tender. Drain the water.

2. Coat a baking sheet using a parchment paper; place salmon fillets on one side. Rub the salmon with 1 Tbsp. of the oil, and sprinkle on ¼ tsp. Black pepper and ¼ tsp. salt. Keep the potatoes next to salmon.

3. With the flat side of a measuring cup, gently crush the potatoes, brush potatoes thoroughly with 1 Tbsp. oil, and drizzle on ¼ tsp. salt, and ¼ tsp. black pepper. Place the pan in the oven and bake for 8 minutes.

4. Remove the pan from the oven and add the haricots verts to the baking sheet to open space. Toss with 2 tsp. oil and ¼ tsp. salt. Put it back in the oven for another 8 minutes. Switch the broiler to high; broil until the salmon and potatoes are browned, about 2 minutes.

5. Combine the red peppers, walnuts, paprika, lemon juice, and the remaining 1/4 tsp. salt and ¼ tsp. In a food processor or blender, add black pepper; blend until smooth.

6. Spoon Romesco over the potatoes and salmon fillets. Garnish with fresh parsley, if needed.

Sesame-Seared Tuna Steaks with Soba Noodles

Swap in booming inflammation-fighting seafood steaks for beef a couple times a week. it takes minutes to prepare.

Serving Size: 4

Prep and Cook Time: 20 min.

Ingredients

- 8 oz. soba (Japanese buckwheat noodles)
- 2 Tbsp. sweet chili sauce
- 1 (6-oz.) bag snow peas
- 2 Tbsp. fresh lime juice
- ¼ cup lower-sodium soy sauce
- 2 Tbsp. light sesame oil
- ¼ cup fresh cilantro leaves
- 1 Tbsp. vegetable oil

- ½ tsp. kosher salt
- 2 Tbsp. white sesame seeds
- 2 Tbsp. black sesame seeds
- 2 (8-oz.) ahi tuna steaks
- Cooking spray
- 2 Tbsp. thinly sliced green onion

Nutrition Information

Per serving: 483 Calories; 16g Fat; 2g Saturated Fat; 40mg Cholesterol; 1342mg Sodium; 49g Carbohydrate; 2g Fiber; 40g Protein; 2g Sugar; 136mg Calcium; 5mg Iron; 7o7mg Potassium

Preparation

1. Cook the soba noodles according to package instructions. Add the snow peas in the final 3 minutes. Rinse with warm water and drain well.

2. Mix the lime juice, soy sauce, chili sauce, and sesame oil in a sizeable bowl; stir well. Add the soba mixture and cilantro; toss to combine.

3. Put the white sesame and black sesame in a shallow dish. Coat the tuna steak with cooking spray and sprinkle with salt evenly. Coat both sides of each steak with sesame seeds and press lightly to make it adhere.

4. Heat the vegetable oil in a large frying pan to medium high. Pour the tuna into the pot; cook for 3 minutes on each side to reach a moderately rare or cooked level. Cut the tuna into thin slices.

5. Divide the soba mixture evenly into four plates. Top with 4 ounces of tuna and garnished with chopped green onion.

Red Curry Chicken and Rice

Mild spices and white rice can be soothing. Spice blends such as curry powder can enhance flavor without adding extra fat, salt or trigger food during ulcers outbreaks. Chopped chicken breasts and peeled cooked potatoes are also easy to digest.

Serving Size: 6

Prep and Cook Time: 40 min.

Ingredients

- 1 Tbsp. curry powder
- 2 Tbsp. extra-virgin olive oil
- 2 tsp. freshly grated ginger
- 1 tsp. paprika

- 1 (14.5-oz.) can diced tomatoes
- 2 cups peeled and cubed Russet potato (from 1 large potato)
- 3 Tbsp. natural peanut butter
- 2 cups lower-sodium vegetable broth
- ¾ tsp. kosher salt
- ½ tsp. black pepper
- 2 cups fresh baby spinach
- 1 ½ cups shredded rotisserie chicken
- 3 cups cooked white rice for serving
- Fresh basil for garnish, if desired
- 1 ½ cups unsweetened refrigerated cashew milk (or 1 can light coconut milk)

Nutrition Information

Per serving: 333 Calories; 11g Fat; 2g Saturated Fat; 32mg Cholesterol; 628mg Sodium; 40g

Carbohydrate; 4g Fiber; 17g Protein; 3g Sugar; 99mg Calcium; 3mg Iron; 538mg Potassium

Preparation

1. Heat oil in a sizeable high-sided skillet over medium heat. Stir in paprika, curry powder and ginger; cook for 2 minutes. Stir in the potatoes and cook for 5 minutes, stirring occasionally, until light golden brown.

2. Add peanut butter, broth, salt and pepper; allow the mixture to boil. Lower the heat to medium-low, and cover the pot until the potatoes are tender, about 20 minutes.

3. Put the spinach and cook until it's wilted, about 2 minutes. Put the chicken and cashew milk; stir to combine, leave uncovered and Simmer for 5 minutes.

4. Put ½ cup rice in each of 6 serving plates and top with 1 cup curry mixture. Serve with fresh basil, if desired.

Moroccan Quinoa-Stuffed Eggplant with Pine-Nut Parmesan

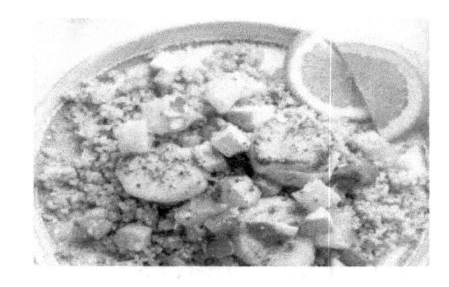

Do not let the mild taste of eggplant fool you. This vegetable is rich in vitamins and minerals. Patients with ulcers are sensitive to lactose, this recipe uses pine nuts and nutritional yeast to make plant-based Parmesan cheese.

Serving Size: 4

Prep and Cook Time: 1 hr.

<u>Ingredients</u>

- 2 medium eggplants
- 3 garlic cloves, minced
- 3 Tbsp. extra-virgin olive oil, divided
- ¾ tsp. kosher salt, divided
- ½ cup dry quinoa
- 1 (14.5-oz.) can diced tomatoes
- 2 Tbsp. mild harissa paste
- 2 cups lower-sodium vegetable broth
- 1 Tbsp. nutritional yeast
- 3 Tbsp. finely chopped pine nuts (or slivered almonds)
- ¼ tsp. garlic powder
- 4 Tbsp. thinly sliced fresh basil leaves

Nutrition Information

Per serving: 331 Calories; 17g Fat; 2g Saturated Fat; 0mg Cholesterol; 734mg Sodium; 39g Carbohydrate; 12g Fiber; 8g Protein; 14g Sugar; 89mg Calcium; 2mg Iron; 1023mg Potassium

Preparation

1. Preheat the oven to 375°F. Cut the eggplant in half along the length of the stem. Cut the flesh of the eggplant into a circle, and then dig out the flesh. Set aside. Place the eggplant half face up on the baking sheet.

2. Brush the eggplant halves with 1 Tbsp. of the olive oil and ¼ tsp of salt. Roast the eggplant for 20 minutes, or until golden brown and lightly tender.

3. At the same time, heat the remaining 2 tablespoons oil in a sizeable frying pan over medium heat. Chop the reserved eggplant flesh and put it in the pot. Cook for 6 to 7 minutes, until tender. Add garlic, harissa, quinoa and teaspoon salt; cook for 2 minutes, stirring often.

4. Add the diced tomatoes and broth, and bring the mixture to a boil. Simmer for a short while, cover the pot and cook for 15 to 20 minutes, until the quinoa is cooked and absorbed most of the liquid.

5. Remove the eggplant halves from the oven and add the quinoa mixture evenly. Place back in the oven for 15 minutes.
6. Mix pine nuts, nutritional yeast, garlic powder, and remaining ¼ tsp salt in a medium bowl. Drizzle Pine Nut Parmesan over each the eggplant half, and serve each with 1 Tbsp. basil.

Chili Shrimp Tacos with Avocado-Tomatillo Sauce

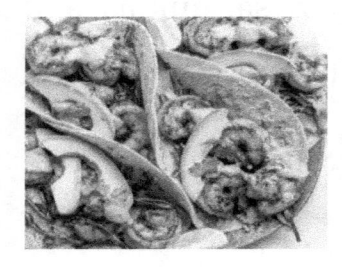

Spice up your tacos with Mediterranean flavor, replace the beef with shrimp. This recipe also contains fiber rich vegetables, which can help feed beneficial intestinal bacteria, thereby helping to control symptoms.

Serving Size: 4

Prep and Cook Time: 25 min.

Ingredients

- 1 lb. medium raw shrimp, peeled and deveined
- ½ tsp. ground cumin
- 1 tsp. chili powder
- 1 tsp. kosher salt, divided
- 1 Tbsp. plus 2 tsp. extra-virgin olive oil, divided
- 6 oz. fresh tomatillos, peeled and halved
- 3 Tbsp. thinly sliced green onion
- 1 Tbsp. fresh lime juice ▪ 1 ripe avocado, divided
- 2 cups shredded red cabbage
- 8 (6-in.) corn tortillas, warmed
- ½ cup fresh cilantro leaves, divided

- ½ medium jalapeño, seeded (optional)

Nutrition Information

Per serving: 344 Calories; 14g Fat; 2g Saturated Fat; 143mg Cholesterol; 670mg Sodium; 33g Carbohydrate; 7g Fiber; 19g Protein; 4g Sugar; 93mg Calcium; 1mg Iron; 589mg Potassium

Preparation

1. Put the shrimp in a small bowl and toss with cumin, chili powder and ½ tsp. salt. Heat 1 Tbsp. oil in a sizeable skillet over medium-high heat.

2. Place the shrimp into the cooking pan and arrange in a single layer, cook for 3 minutes. Turn other side and cook additional 2 minutes. Transfer to a bowl; keep warm.

3. To Prepare the Avocado-Tomatillo sauce, mix ½ of the avocado, ¼ cup cilantro, jalapeño (optional), tomatillos and remaining ½ tsp. salt in a blender; blend until smooth.

4. Put cabbage, remaining ¼ cup cilantro, lime juice, remaining 2 tsp. oil, green onion and ¼ tsp. salt in a bowl; toss to combine.

5. Distribute the shrimp and cabbage mixture equally between warmed tortillas. Each taco is topped with 2 Tbsp. Avocado-Tomatillo Sauce. Slice and garnish with remaining ½ avocado.

Chicken Piccata Pasta

This dinner is perfect for special occasions and is fast enough to take a dip in a working day. Compared with most Piccata pasta, this pasta can reduce the butter content to keep saturated fat at a low level (a large amount of fat can trigger the occurrence of ulcerative colitis). Enhance specificity and increase

Serving Size: 4

Prep and Cook Time: 25 min.

Ingredients

- 3 Tbsp. extra-virgin olive oil
- 10 oz. dry angel hair pasta
- 1 Tbsp. minced fresh garlic (or a tsp. if you're sensitive)
- ¼ cup brined capers, drained
- ⅓ cup chopped fresh parsley
- 3 Tbsp. unsalted butter, divided
- 1 lb. skinless, boneless chicken breasts, butterflied and then cut in half
- ½ tsp. kosher salt
- ¾ tsp. black pepper, divided
- 3 Tbsp. all-purpose flour
- ½ cup dry white wine

- 1 cup lower-sodium chicken broth
- 2 Tbsp. fresh lemon juice

Nutrition Information

Per serving: 623 Calories; 25g Fat; 8g Saturated Fat; 106mg Cholesterol; 519mg Sodium; 59g Carbohydrate; 3g Fiber; 37g Protein; 3g Sugar; 39mg Calcium; 3mg Iron; 617mg Potassium

Preparation

1. According to package directions, cook the pasta in boiling salted water until hardened. Drain the water and transfer to a plate.

2. Heat oil and 2 Tbsp. butter at the same time in the large frying pan over medium-high heat. Season the chicken with salt and ½ tsp. black pepper.

3. Sprinkle flour evenly and shake off excess flour. Add the chicken to the frying pan and cook without disturbing for 3 minutes per side, until golden brown. Transfer to a plate.

4. Pour the garlic into the pot; cook for 1 minute, stirring constantly. Add wine; cook for 2 minutes, scrape the brown bits from the pan, until halved. Stir in the broth, lemon juice, capers and the remaining teaspoon. Black pepper. Put the chicken back in the pot and simmer for 5 minutes.

5. Remove the chicken from the pot and place it on the pasta. Add the remaining 1 tbsp. butter into the pan and stir vigorously to mix.

6. Drizzle sauce over chicken and pasta. Serve with fresh parsley.

Note: Garlic is a high-FODMAP

Balsamic-Roasted Salmon with Artichoke Gremolata

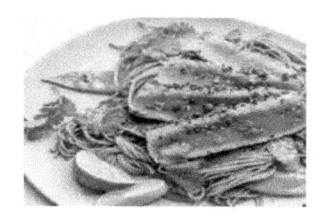

This dish is restaurant-worthy, a cinch to make, and packed with ingredients that are ulcers remission-friendly. For good reason, salmon is considered a super food: it is a rich source of vitamin D, which can help quench inflammation in the intestines.

Serving Size: 4

Prep and Cook Time: 50 min.

Ingredients

- 4 (6-oz.) salmon fillets
- ½ tsp. kosher salt
- 2 Tbsp. balsamic vinegar
- 3 Tbsp. extra-virgin olive oil, divided
- 2 tsp. Dijon mustard

- 2 tsp. honey
- ¾ cup halved cherry tomatoes
- ½ cup canned artichoke hearts in brine, finely chopped
- 1 Tbsp. finely chopped pine nuts (or raw slivered almonds)
- 2 cups fresh spinach
- 1 garlic clove, minced
- 1 Tbsp. fresh lemon juice
- 2 Tbsp. fresh chopped parsley
- ½ tsp. black pepper
- 2 cups lower-sodium vegetable broth
- 1 ⅓ cup dry pearl couscous

Nutrition Information

Per serving: 634 Calories; 23g Fat; 3g Saturated Fat; 94mg Cholesterol; 534mg Sodium; 64g Carbohydrate; 4g Fiber; 44g Protein; 7g Sugar; 68mg Calcium; 3mg Iron; 912mg Potassium

Preparation

1. In a wide-rimmed bowl, put the salmon and season with salt. Mix 1 tbsp. oil, vinegar, mustard, and honey in a medium sized bowl turn with a whisk. Set aside 2 tbsp., pour the remaining mixture over the salmon and leave to stand for 15 minutes.

2. In the meantime, combine the artichokes, pine nuts, garlic, lemon juice, black pepper, parsley, and the remaining 2 Tbsp. olive oil in a bowl; blend well. Only set aside.

3. In a medium saucepan, bring the broth to a boil. Add couscous, lower the heat to a simmer, cover and cook for around 15 minutes until tender. Remove from the heat and stir in the tomatoes and spinach. Cover to keep warm.

4. Preheat the oven to 450°F. Insert the salmon on a baking sheet lined with foil and bake it for 8 minutes. Remove from the oven and brush with reserved marinade; put back in the oven, and bake for additional 5 minutes.

5. Divide the couscous mixture equally into 4 bowls each. Serve each bowl with 1 salmon fillet and 2 Tbsp. artichoke gremolata.

Mild spices and white rice satisfy and help relax. Any time stomach ulcers symptoms flare up, serve this comforting dish.

Roasted Asparagus with Caper Dressing

Roasting will thicken the grassy taste of asparagus; caper sauce provides saltiness. Serve with grilled fish or meat.

Prep and Cook time: 40 minutes

Ingredients:

- 2 bunches of asparagus (about 2 pounds)
- 1 tablespoon plus 2 teaspoons extra virgin olive oil, separated.
- ¼ teaspoons salt and fresh pepper, separated (optional)
- 2 Cups of chopped scallions, cupped parsley leaves,
- 3 tablespoons of rinsed capers (on-line packaging and salt-packed capers in gourmet stores)
- 2 tablespoons of white wine vinegar (optional)

Preparation:

1. Preheat the oven to 450°F. Trim the hard ends of the asparagus; place on a baking sheet.

2. Sprinkle 1 tablespoon of oil, salt and teaspoon pepper (if needed) on the asparagus; toss the coat.

3. Spread out a layer and roast, rotating once halfway, until the asparagus starts to soften and brown (12 to 14 minutes).

4. Transfer to serving plate. At the same time, put the shallots, coriander, capers, vinegar (if needed), the remaining 2 teaspoons of oil and teaspoon of pepper (if needed) into the blender and blend well until the ingredients are chopped or flattened. Serve asparagus with seasoning.

Butternut Squash Soup with Lemongrass

Abdominal healing is improved by using this soothing low FODMAP soup. Peeled, cooked and mixed vegetables are easy to digest during ulcer attacks.

Preparation time: 1 hour

Ingredients:

- 2 tablespoons of extra virgin olive oil

- 4 of cups peeled and cubed butternut squash
- 2½ cups of chopped carrots (about 3 large carrots)
- 1½ tablespoon of chopped fresh ginger
- 1 tablespoon of lemongrass sauce
- 1 teaspoon of turmeric powder
- ½ tablespoon of kosher salt
- 4 cups of low-sodium vegetable broth.
- ½ cup plus 4 tablespoons of coconut-milk yogurt, separately.
- light green vegetables or fresh basil for garnish (optional)

Preparation:

1. Heat oil in a Dutch oven or large stockpot in a medium heat. Add squash and carrots; cook for 7 minutes, stirring occasionally, until light golden brown.

2. Stir in ginger, lemongrass paste, turmeric and salt; cook for 2 minutes, until fragrant. Add

broth and increase heat until the mixture boils. Then reduce the heat to a low level.

3. Cover the pot and cook for about 40 to 45 minutes, until the vegetables are tender.

4. Carefully pour the mixture into the blender; add a cup of yogurt. Remove the central part of the blender cover to allow steam to escape, fix the cover on the blender. Put a clean towel on the opening of the lid. Processing until smooth.
5. Divide soup evenly into several bowls. Add yogurt into each serving, and garnish with fresh basil or microgreens, (if needed).

Fried Rice with Miso-Turmeric Vinaigrette

The fiber content of white rice is lower than brown rice, so when your ulcer symptoms occur, white rice is easier to digest.

Preparation time: 40 minutes

Ingredients:

- 2 tablespoons of unseasoned rice vinegar
- 2 teaspoons of sesame oil (unbaked)
- 2 teaspoons of white miso sauce
- 1 teaspoon of salt
- ½ tablespoon of freshly grated ginger
- 2 tablespoons of turmeric powder
- 2 cups vegetable oil
- 2 cups of roughly chopped cabbage Choy
- 1 cup matchstick carrots
- 3 cups cooked white rice
- 2 tablespoons of low-sodium soy sauce
- 3 large eggs, whisked
- 2 tablespoons of eggs
- 2 tablespoons of chopped fresh basil

Preparation:

1. Combine vinegar, sesame oil, mio, ginger and turmeric in a small bowl, prepare the seasoning; stir with whisk. Set aside.

2. Heat the vegetable oil in a large pot to medium high. Add cabbage and carrots; cook for 5 minutes, stirring often, until soft. Add the rice and soy sauce, and then press the rice evenly into the frying pan. Cook for about three minutes until the rice starts to become crispy. Toss and combine.

3. By pushing the rice and vegetables to all sides, a large opening is created in the center of the pot. Pour in the eggs and keep stirring until the eggs are disrupted (about 1 to 2 minutes).

4. Mix the eggs and rice well, and stir in the basil. Place the fried rice evenly between the some plates.
   Top with drizzle turmeric balsamic vinegar

Red Curry Chicken and Rice

Soft Spice blends like curry powder boost taste without adding extra fat, salt, or trigger foods during a ulcers flare. Crushed chicken breast and peeled, cooked potato is also easy on digestion.

Serving Size: 6

Prep and Cook Time: 40 min.

Ingredients
- 2 Tbsp. extra-virgin olive oil
- 1 Tbsp. curry powder
- 2 cups lower-sodium vegetable broth

- 2 tsp. freshly grated ginger
- 1 tsp. paprika
- 2 cups peeled and cubed Russet potato (from 1 large potato)
- 3 Tbsp. natural peanut butter
- 1 (14.5-oz.) can diced tomatoes
- ¾ tsp. kosher salt
- ½ tsp. black pepper
- 2 cups fresh baby spinach
- 1 ½ cups shredded rotisserie chicken
- 3 cups cooked white rice for serving
- 1 ½ cups unsweetened refrigerated cashew milk (or 1 can light coconut milk)
- Fresh basil for garnish, if desired

Nutrition Information

Per serving: 323 Calories; 11g Fat; 2g Saturated Fat; 32mg Cholesterol; 628mg Sodium; 40g Carbohydrate; 4g Fiber; 17g Protein; 3g Sugar; 99mg Calcium; 3mg Iron; 518mg Potassium

Preparation

1. Heat oil to medium in a big, high-sided skillet. Insert curry powder, paprika, and ginger; cook for 2 minutes. Stir in the potatoes and cook for 5 minutes, stirring occasionally, until golden brown. Insert peanut butter, broth, tomatoes, salt, and pepper; bring the mixture to a boil.

2. Reduce to medium-low and simmer, covered, for about 20 minutes, or until the potato is tender. Stir in the spinach and cook for about 2 minutes, until wilted. Add the cashew milk and chicken; stir to mix. for 5 minutes, uncovered.

3. Put ½ cup rice in each of 6 bowls, top with 1 cup curry mixture. Serve with fresh basil, if needed.

Simple Roast Chicken

No reason to make a fuss about complicated techniques to obtain delicious, rich and simple roast chicken, which is the ultimate comfort food.

Preparation time: 1 hour

Ingredients:

- 1 small onion, peeled and sliced into thin slices
- 3 cloves of garlic, peeled and sliced into slices
- 1 5 pounds of chicken, guts removed crushed
- 3 sprigs of fresh tarragon (substitution: teaspoon powder)
- 2 tablespoons of extra virgin olive oil, 1 teaspoon kosher salt,
- ½ teaspoon of freshly ground pepper (optional)

Preparation:

1. Preheat the oven to 375°F. Put onion, garlic, tarragon and thyme into the chicken cavity. Tie the legs with kitchen rope together, closing the opening of the cavity.

2. Pull the wings so that the tip overlaps the top of the breast; tie them in place, and wrap the wings and body with rope.

3. Rub the chicken with oil, salt and pepper (if needed). Place on a baking tray with breasts facing down.

4. Roast the chicken for about 25 minutes. Place the breasts face up and continue to bake. Baste occasionally with the pan juice until the thermometer is inserted into the thickest part of the thigh without touching the bones records 175°F per 1 hour.

5. Transfer the roast chicken to cutting board; rest for 10 minutes. Remove the strings before carving.

Roasting techniques:

- Very cold meat will not be grilled evenly. Place it on the counter while the oven is preheating. Durable cotton kitchen lines are sold in kitchenware stores most gourmet markets and large supermarkets. Do not use sewing thread or yarn that may contain inedible dyes or unpleasant chemicals.

- Heavy-duty, high-side bake ware is essential to evenly conduct heat. Never replace the cookie table. When baking, the internal temperature of the oven will increase by about 10 degrees. Natural juices will also be re-incorporated into the fiber of the meat, the skin or crusty will dry out a bit to make the dinner more toothy and fleshy.

Oven-Poached Salmon Fillets

Baking salmon fillets can produce a moisturizing effect as long as you remember the two basic rules of fish cooking: choose only the freshest Fish, don't overcook it. If needed, sprinkle your favorite sauce on top.

Preparation time: 30 minutes

Ingredients:

- 1 pound salmon fillet, cut into 4 portions, peeled,
- 2 tablespoons of dry white wine if needed (substitute: broth).
- ½ teaspoon of salt and fresh pepper to taste (optional)
- 2 tablespoons chopped green onions, (1 medium)

Preparation:

1. Preheat the oven to 425°F. Apply cooking spray.

2. On a 9-inch glass bakeware or an 8-inch glass bakeware. Place the skinless side of the salmon in the prepared pan.

3. Sprinkle with wine or broth. Season with salt and pepper (if needed), then sprinkle with shallots.

4. Cover with foil and bake until the center salmon is opaque, then start to peel, for 15 to 25 minutes, depending on the thickness.

5. After the salmon is ready, transfer to the plate. Remove all the liquid remaining in the salmon pot.

Salmon chowder

Salmon chowder flavor can makes the meal delicious by adding dill or tarragon. Each herb can give the soup a unique flavor.

Preparation time: 45 minutes

Ingredients:

- 1 tablespoon of canola oil
- 1 cup of chopped carrots
- 1 chopped celery cup (optional)
- 4 cups of low-sodium chicken broth (check the ingredients on the label)
- 1½ cups of water
- 1 ounce of 12 ounces of peeled salmon fillet, preferably caught in the wild.
- 2 cups of frozen cauliflower florets, thawed and chopped (optional)
- 3 tablespoons of chopped fresh chives or spring onions (substitute: teaspoon Onion powder)
- 1 cup of instant mashed potatoes.

- 2 teaspoons of dried tarragon (substitute: to 1 teaspoon of powder)
- 1 tablespoon of Dijon mustard (optional).
- ½ teaspoon of salt
- Freshly ground pepper to taste (optional)

Preparation:

1. Heat oil in a large pot or Dutch oven over medium heat. Add carrots and celery (if needed) and cook, stirring often, until the vegetables start to turn brown for 3-4 minutes.

2. Add the broth, water, salmon, broccoli (if needed) and chives or spring onions, then simmer on low heat.

3. Cover the pot and cook, keeping it mild, until the salmon is cooked for 5-8 minutes. Move the salmon to a clean cutting board. Use a fork to peel it into bite-sized pieces.

4. Stir the potato chips (or remaining mashed potatoes), dill or tarragon and mustard sauce (if needed) into the soup until well combined.
5. Add salmon and reheat. Season with salt and pepper (if needed).

Warm Chicken Sausage & Potato Salad

This warm bistro-style salad is the perfect dish to share with guests at the next dinner party.

Preparation time: 45 minutes

Ingredients:

- 1 pound small potatoes cut in half
- 1 5-ounce bag of arugula (about 4 cups, lightly packed)) (substitute: spinach)
- 12 ounces of precooked chicken sausage cut crosswise into ½-inch pieces (check ingredients on the label)
- 1 cup of cider vinegar (optional)
- 1 tablespoon of maple syrup (optional)

- 1 tablespoon of whole-grain or Dijon mustard (optional)
- 1 tablespoon of extra virgin olive oil and fresh pepper to taste (optional)

Preparation:

1. Pour an inch of water to a boil in a Dutch oven. Put the potatoes in a steamer and cover with steam until they are cooked for about 15 minutes.

2. Transfer to a large bowl and add arugula or spinach; cover with foil to keep warm. Cook the sausage in average heat, stir often, until it turns brown and heat for about 5 minutes, then add the arugula into the potatoes mixture.

3. Remove the pot from the heat and whisk in the vinegar (if needed), maple syrup (if needed) and mustard (if needed), scraping off any brown crumbs.

4. Stir gradually in the oil. Pour the seasoning over the salad until the arugula is wilted. Season with pepper (if needed).

Curried Carrot & Apple

This colorful soup is simple and delicious. Use apples that cook easily and soft. Mackintosh is great.

Preparation time: 1 hour

Ingredients:

- 1 tablespoon of extra virgin olive oil
- 1 large onion, chopped (2 cups)
- 1 celery stalk, chopped (optional) 1 tablespoon curry powder (substitute: turmeric powder)
- 5 large carrots, peeled and thinly sliced (3 Cup)
- 2 large McIntosh or other apples, peeled and chopped (3 cups)
- 1 bay leaf
- ½ teaspoon of salt

fresh pepper to taste (optional)

1 tablespoon chopped fresh parsley, dill or basil for garnish (optional)

<u>Preparation</u>:

1. Heat oil in a large pot or medium stock pot over medium heat.

2. Stir the onion and celery (if needed); cook until the onion is soft and translucent, for4 –5 minutes; not brown.

3. Add curry powder or turmeric. Then add carrots, apples and bay leaves. Stir well over medium heat for 2 minutes, and then add broth and salt.

4. Bring the mixture to a boil, by reducing the heat. Cover the pan tightly and simmer for 15 - 20 minutes, until the carrots and apples are soft.

5. Take out the bay leaves. Use a tablespoon to transfer the soup solids to a food processor, add about cup of broth; process into a smooth slurry. Pour the puree into the soup.

6. Reheat and season with pepper (if needed). Serve piping hot food and sprinkle each serving with fresh herbs if you want.

Sweet Potato and Lentil Soup

When your ulcer is in remission, legumes (such as lentils) can provide you with the ideal fiber and protein dosage.

Preparation time: 50 minutes

Ingredients:

- 2 tablespoons of extra virgin olive oil
- 1 cup of chopped yellow onions
- 3 garlic cloves
- 2 tablespoons of tomato paste
- 2 teaspoons of cumin powder
- 2 tablespoons of Garam masala
- 1 large sweet potato, peeled and cut into thin slices. Fragments (about 2 cups)
- 1 cup uncooked brown lentils

- 4 cups low-sodium vegetable soup
- 2 cups water
- 1 (14.5 ounces) can roast tomatoes
- 1 teaspoon of kosher salt
- 1 bunch of kale, stalks removed and chopped fresh parsley for garnish (optional)

Preparation:

1. Heat the oil to medium in a large saucepan or Dutch oven. Add onions; cook for 5 minutes, until tender. Add garlic, tomato paste, cumin and Garam Masala; cook for 2 minutes, stirring occasionally.

2. Add sweet potatoes; stir and cook for 5 minutes. Add the lentils, add the stock, water, tomatoes and salt; bring the mixture to a boil.

3. Reduce the heat, simmer on low heat, and cover, until the lentils are cooked and the sweet potatoes are tender, about 30 to 35 minutes.

4. Pour in the kale and stir and cook until the kale is wilted for about 2 minutes. Divide evenly into several bowls. You can garnish with fresh parsley (If needed).

Zucchini Noodles with Ginger-Peanut Sauce

This delicious lunch is also low in FODMAP and low carb, which is especially important for ulcer patients on steroids.

Preparation time: 30 minutes

Ingredients:

- 3 tablespoons of natural creamy peanut butter
- 2 tablespoons low-sodium soy sauce
- 1½ teaspoon of fresh ginger juice
- 2 teaspoons of lime
- 2 tablespoons of pure extra virgin olive oil, separately
- 1 ounce (14 ounces), drain the firm tofu cubes, drain, pat dry, and cut into 1-inch pieces
- ½ teaspoon of kosher salt
- 1½ cup of matchstick carrots
- 1 red sweet pepper, thinly sliced
- 4 medium zucchini, thinly sliced and spiraled into thin noodles

Preparation:

1. In a small bowl, combine the peanut butter, soy sauce, ginger, lime juice and maple syrup

and mix well. Set aside. Heat a tablespoon of olive oil in a nonstick pan.

2. Add tofu; cook until the tofu is golden and crisp, stirring occasionally. Season the tofu with a small spoon. Salt; transfer to a plate. Season with the remaining ¼ teaspoon of salt.

3. Put the zucchini noodles in the pot; cook for 2 to 3 minutes, turning frequently to heat, but not fully cooked. Add tofu and half of the peanut butter to the frying pan.

4. Place the zucchini noodle mixture evenly between some plates. Drizzle the remaining peanut butter on top.

Snacks and Desserts Recipes

Cherry Almond-Butter Bars

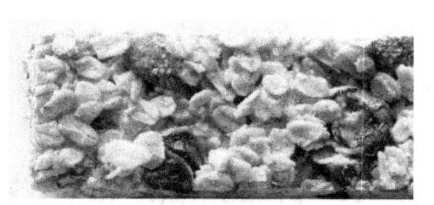

These protein and fiber-packed bars beat the packed bars every day of the week. Who knew you could get an increase in calcium from almonds and pecans? This is a big advantage for people with stomach ulcers who are often deficient in minerals. These bars also provide heart-healthy fat and dietary fiber.

Serving Size: 10

Prep and Cook Time: 35 min.

Ingredients

- ¾ cup creamy almond butter
- 1 tsp. vanilla extract
- ½ tsp. kosher salt
- ⅓ cup pecans
- 1 egg white, whisked
- 2 cups old-fashioned oats
- ¼ cup pure maple syrup
- ½ cup chopped dried cherries

Nutrition Information

Per serving: 243 Calories; 14g Fat; 2g Saturated Fat; 0mg Cholesterol; 147mg Sodium; 27g Carbohydrate; 5g Fiber; 7g Protein; 11g Sugar; 95mg Calcium; 2mg Iron; 258mg Potassium

Preparation

1. Preheat the oven to 350°F. Arrange an 8x8-inch square baking pan with parchment paper.

2. Mix the almond butter, vanilla, maple syrup, salt and egg white in a large bowl; stir to combine. Stir in the oats, cherries and pistachios, then transfer the mixture to the prepared baking pan. Use a spatula to press the mixture firmly into the pan.

3. Bake for 20 minutes, or until it turns light brown. Allow it cool completely before removing it from the pan using parchment paper. Place on a cutting board and cut into 10 bars.

Strawberry-Banana Nice Cream

Homemade ice cream will not cause abdominal pain. When the colon is stimulated, bananas are easy to digest, and the potassium content in bananas is high, which is one of the electrolytes lost in diarrhea caused by flare.

Serving Size: 2

Prep and Cook Time: 10 min.

Ingredients

- 1 cup frozen strawberries
- 1 ½ medium frozen bananas, chopped
- 3 Tbsp. unsweetened vanilla almond milk

Nutrition Information

Per serving: 107 Calories; 1g Fat; 0g Saturated Fat; 0mg Cholesterol; 19mg Sodium; 27g Carbohydrate; 4g Fiber; 1g Protein; 14g Sugar; 35mg Calcium; 1mg Iron; 425mg Potassium

Preparation

Mix all ingredients in a high-power mixer. Blend until creamy, stop and scrape off the sides as needed. Enjoy immediately or spread out in a bread pan, freeze for another 30 minutes, then remove with an ice cream scoop.

Chocolate-Avocado Mousse

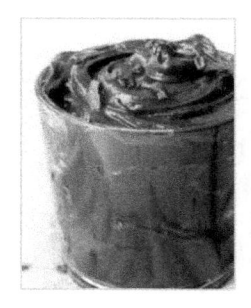

The healthy ingredients of this mousse incorporate a nutritious and easily tolerated avocado, which is also an important source of potassium. A dessert you that can make you feel better when you have ulcer flare; it's dairy-free with healthy fats.

Serving Size: 4

Prep and Cook Time: 1 hr. 10 min.

Ingredients

- 2 large ripe avocados
- ¼ cup pure maple syrup
- ¼ cup regular unsweetened cocoa powder
- 1 tsp. vanilla extract
- 2 Tbsp. dark baking cocoa
- 3 Tbsp. unsweetened cashew milk (or unsweetened almond, coconut, or soy milk)
- ¼ tsp. sea salt
- Fresh raspberries for garnish (optional)

Nutrition Information

Per serving: 212 Calories; 16g Fat; 3g Saturated Fat; 0mg Cholesterol; 190mg Sodium; 27g Carbohydrate; 9g Fiber; 4g Protein; 13g Sugar; 44mg Calcium; 1mg Iron; 623mg Potassium

Preparation

Put all ingredients (except raspberries) in a high-power blender or food processor; blend until smooth. Transfer to a bowl and let cool for 1 hour. Divide into four bowls; top with the raspberries.

Rosemary Roasted-Chickpea Snack Mix

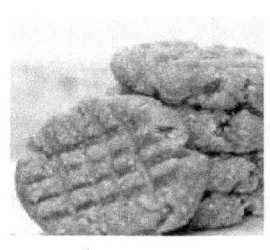

Chickpeas contain fiber, protein and a lot of nutrients. Chickpeas are small power plants of protein and fiber, exactly what you want in a snack.

Serving Size: 6

Prep and Cook Time: 1 hr.

Ingredients

- 1 tsp. kosher salt
- 1 (15-oz.) can chickpeas, drained, rinsed, and patted dried
- ½ cup chopped toasted walnuts

- 1 Tbsp. extra-virgin olive oil
- ½ cup chopped dried apricots
- 1 Tbsp. finely chopped fresh rosemary
- ½ tsp. garlic powder
- ¼ tsp. cayenne pepper

Nutrition Information

Per serving: 204 Calories; 10g Fat; 1g Saturated Fat; 0mg Cholesterol; 473mg Sodium; 25g Carbohydrate; 6g Fiber; 7g Protein; 7g Sugar; 52mg Calcium; 1mg Iron; 124mg Potassium

Preparation

1. Preheat the oven to 400°F. Mix the chickpeas with oil, rosemary, salt, garlic powder and cayenne.

2. Arrange on a framed baking sheet and bake for 45 minutes, or until golden brown and crispy, toss once halfway through. Let it cool on a baking sheet for 10 minutes, then transfer to a bowl.

3. Add walnuts and apricots to the chickpeas; toss up. Store at room temperature in a closed container for up to 5 days.

Peanut-Butter Cookie-Dough Bites

This treat provides good protein without being overly sweet. During a ulcer outbreak, smaller, more frequent meals and snacks are usually best. These bites provide enough energy to help you through the difficult times.

Serving Size: 10

Prep and Cook Time: 15 min.

Ingredients
- 1 ¾ cups old-fashioned rolled oats
- ¼ cup pure maple syrup
- 1 cup natural peanut butter
- 1 tsp. vanilla extract
- ½ tsp. ground cinnamon
- ½ tsp. kosher salt

Nutrition Information

Per serving: 223 Calories; 14g Fat; 2g Saturated Fat; 0mg Cholesterol; 181mg Sodium; 20g Carbohydrate; 3g Fiber; 7g Protein; 6g Sugar; 17mg Calcium; 1mg Iron; 72mg Potassium

Preparation

1. Place the oats in the food processor; process until thoroughly chopped.

2. Transfer to a large bowl and add the remaining ingredients; stir to combine.

3. Use a cookie scoop to make the mixture into 20-22 bites, or roll into small balls. Store in an airtight container and refrigerate for up to 2 weeks.

Raspberry-Oat Streusel Bars

Maintaining a stable gastrointestinal tract is important to prevent symptoms of stomach ulcers. These bars contain fiber from whole grains and berries, which feed beneficial gut bacteria and help maintain a healthy intestinal wall. These snack bars can be prepared in just 15 minutes. They are also delicious!

Serving Size: 16

Prep and Cook Time: 1 hr.

Ingredients

- 2 cups fresh raspberries
- Cooking spray
- 3 Tbsp. pure maple syrup
- 2 Tbsp. corn starch
- 5 Tbsp unsalted butter, melted
- 1 ½ cups old-fashioned rolled oats
- 1 cup white whole-wheat flour
- 1 tsp. vanilla extract
- ¾ cup coconut sugar (or brown sugar)
- ¾ tsp. kosher salt
- 3 Tbsp. extra-virgin olive oil

Nutrition Information

Per serving: 164 Calories; 7g Fat; 2g Saturated Fat; 10mg Cholesterol; 91mg Sodium; 24g Carbohydrate; 3g Fiber; 2g Protein; 12g Sugar; 18mg Calcium; 1mg Iron; 63mg Potassium

Preparation

1. Mix the maple syrup, raspberries, cornstarch and 3 tablespoons of water in a medium pot. Simmer and mash the berries to break them down. Reduce the heat to medium-low level; cook until thick, for about 5 minutes. Remove from the heat and let cool slightly.

2. Preheat the oven to 350°F. Coat an 11" x 7" baking pan with cooking spray. In a medium bowl, Mix the oats, salt, coconut sugar and flour. Add butter, oil and vanilla. Reserve a ⅔ cup of oatmeal mixture.

3. Sprinkle the remaining oat mixture evenly on the prepared plate; press firmly. Spread the raspberry mixture evenly on top, and then sprinkle the remaining oat mixture on the

raspberries. Bake for about 35 minutes until it turns light brown.

4. Cool completely on the wire rack. Cut into 16 squares. Store in an airtight container for up to 3 days.

No-Bake Brownie Bites

If you are a fan of Nutella, you will love the chocolate hazelnut flavor in these energy snacks. When you have stomach ulcers, limiting sugar supplementation is an important way to stop inflammation. These bites are naturally sweetened by dates and also increase the concentrated dose of fiber, vitamins and minerals.

Serving Size: 10

Prep and Cook Time: 15 min.

Ingredients

- 12 pitted Medjool dates
- ½ cup raw cashews
- 2 Tbsp. cocoa powder
- ¼ cup almond butter
- ½ cup hazelnuts
- ½ tsp. vanilla extract
- ¼ tsp. kosher salt
-

Nutrition Information

Per serving: 183 Calories; 10g Fat; 1g Saturated Fat; 0mg Cholesterol; 70mg Sodium; 23g Carbohydrate; 4g Fiber; 4g Protein; 17g Sugar; 47mg Calcium; 1mg Iron; 214mg Potassium

Preparation

1. Put the dates, hazelnuts and cashews in a food processor; process until mixture is finely chopped. Add vanilla, almond butter, cocoa

powder, and salt; process until mixture just starts to clump together.

2. Roll the mixture into 1 Tbsp. balls and chill until ready to serve. Store in an airtight container in the refrigerator for up to 14 days.

Cucumber and Tuna-Salad Sushi Rolls

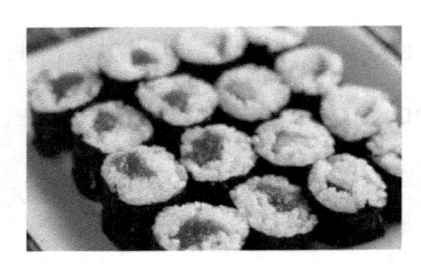

Use pop-up high-protein snacks between meals to keep you energized. When you need some fillings that will not cause harm, you can choose this snack. Cucumber has the lowest fiber content and high-water content, so it is easy to digest. During ulcers outbreaks, tuna will provide you with a healthy protein dose to make you satisfied.

Serving Size: 1

Prep and Cook Time: 15 min.

Ingredients

- 1 (3-oz.) pouch wild albacore tuna, drained
- 2 tsp. mayonnaise
- ½ tsp. Dijon mustard
- ¼ tsp. kosher salt
- ¼ tsp. lemon zest, plus 1 tsp. fresh lemon juice
- ¼ tsp. black pepper
- 1 English cucumber, halved crosswise

Nutrition Information

Per serving: 200 Calories; 8g Fat; 1g Saturated Fat; 41mg Cholesterol; 874mg Sodium; 7g Carbohydrate; 3g Fiber; 30g Protein; 41g Sugar; 64mg Calcium; 1mg Iron; 418mg Potassium

Preparation

1. Put the tuna, lemon zest, juice, mustard, salt, mayonnaise and pepper in bowl; mix well.

2. Trim off cucumber ends; reserve for another use. Slice cucumber halves lengthwise into 10 ⅛-inch-thick ribbons using any slicer. Place the slices flat on a cutting board.

3. Sprinkle 2 tsp. of the tuna mixture towards one end of each cucumber ribbon, about 1 inch from the edge. Wrap edge of each cucumber ribbon over tuna and continue to roll into sushi-sized bites.

Banana-Chia Pudding

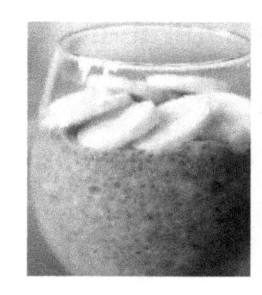

Chia seeds are one of the richest plant sources of ALA (a type of omega-3 fatty acid) and help fight inflammation caused by diseases such as stomach ulcers. Adding bananas to the pudding can provide prebiotic fiber to promote intestinal health.

Serving Size: 2

Prep and Cook Time: 6 hr. 10 min.

Ingredients

- 2 small ripe bananas, divided
- 1 Tbsp. pure maple syrup
- 4 Tbsp. chia seeds
- 1 Tbsp. unsweetened cocoa powder
- 4 Tbsp. chopped walnuts
- 1 cup unsweetened vanilla almond milk
- 2 Tbsp. cacao nibs

Nutrition Information

Per serving: 326 Calories; 7g Fat; 5g Saturated Fat; 0mg Cholesterol; 97mg Sodium; 50g Carbohydrate; 15g Fiber; 9g Protein; 21g Sugar; 266mg Calcium; 4mg Iron; 620mg Potassium

Preparation

1. Put a banana in a bowl and mash it thoroughly with a fork. Transfer to a glass bottle, add Chia seeds, maple syrup, cocoa powder and almond milk. Close the lid and shake to combine. Let stand for 5 minutes, remove cover and stir with a spoon to break clumps. Cover and refrigerate overnight, or at least 6 hours.

2. Pour the chia pudding equally in two bowls. Cut the remaining bananas into thin slices and divide into the two bowls. Garnish each with 2 tablespoons of chopped walnuts and a tablespoon of cocoa nibs.

It's OK to try any of these recipes severally, at any convenient time. They are totally healthy and delicious. The listed ingredients are essential; they will help to heal and improve your inflammation. You can exclude any of the ingredients if it causes discomfort in your body. Enjoy!